Obstetrics and Gynecology

Editor

ELYSE WATKINS

PHYSICIAN ASSISTANT CLINICS

www.physicianassistant.theclinics.com

Consulting Editors
KIM ZUBER
JANE S. DAVIS

July 2022 • Volume 7 • Number 3

ELSEVIER

1600 John F. Kennedy Boulevard • Suite 1800 • Philadelphia, Pennsylvania, 19103-2899

http://www.theclinics.com

PHYSICIAN ASSISTANT CLINICS Volume 7, Number 3
July 2022 ISSN 2405-7991, ISBN-13: 978-0-323-85021-6

Editor: Katerina Heidhausen
Developmental Editor: Axell Ivan Jade Purificacion

Physician Assistant Clinics (ISSN: 2405–7991) is published quarterly by Elsevier Inc., 360 Park Avenue South, New York, NY 10010-1710. Months of issue are January, April, July, and October. Periodicals postage paid at New York, NY and additional mailing offices. Subscription prices are $150.00 per year (US individuals), $305.00 (US institutions), $100.00 (US students), $150.00 (Canadian individuals), $320.00 (Canadian institutions), $100.00 (Canadian students), $150.00 (international individuals), $320.00 (international institutions), and $100.00 (international students). Foreign air speed delivery is included in all *Clinics* subscription prices. All prices are subject to change without notice. POSTMASTER: Send address changes to *Physician Assistant Clinics*, Elsevier Periodicals Customer Service, 11830 Westline Industrial Drive, St. Louis, MO 63146. Customer Service Health Sciences Division, Subscription Customer Service, 3251 Riverport Lane, Maryland Heights, MO 63043. **Customer Service: 1-800-654-2452 (U.S. and Canada); 314-447-8871 (outside U.S. and Canada). Fax: 314-447-8029. E-mail: journalscustomerservice-usa@elsevier.com (for print support); journalsonlinesupport-usa@elsevier.com (for online support).**

Reprints. For copies of 100 or more, of articles in this publication, please contact the Commercial Reprints Department, Elsevier Inc., 360 Park Avenue South, New York, NY 10010-1710. Tel. 212-633-3874; Fax: 212-633-3820; E-mail: reprints@elsevier.com.

Physician Assistant Clinics is covered in *EMBASE/Excerpta Medica* and *ESCI*.

PROGRAM OBJECTIVE

The goal of the *Physician Assistant Clinics* is to keep practicing physician assistants up to date with current clinical practice by providing timely articles reviewing the state of the art in patient care.

TARGET AUDIENCE

Physician Assistants and other healthcare professionals

LEARNING OBJECTIVES

Upon completion of this activity, participants will be able to:

1. Review the strategies used to deliver effective provider-patient communication, including the use of technology-enabled communication tools, in promoting patient engagement, patient safety, honest communication, and positive patient outcomes.
2. Discuss the advantages of effective provider-patient communication among providers, patients, healthcare systems, and communities.
3. Recognize the factors that contribute to the challenges and barriers to effective provider-patient communication.

ACCREDITATION

The Elsevier Office of Continuing Medical Education (EOCME) is accredited by the Accreditation Council for Continuing Medical Education (ACCME) to provide continuing medical education for physicians.

The EOCME designates this journal-based CME activity for a maximum of 13 *AMA PRA Category 1 Credit*(s)™. Physicians should claim only the credit commensurate with the extent of their participation in the activity.

All other health care professionals requesting continuing education credit for this enduring material will be issued a certificate of participation.

DISCLOSURE OF CONFLICTS OF INTEREST

The EOCME assesses conflict of interest with its instructors, faculty, planners, and other individuals who are in a position to control the content of CME activities. All relevant conflicts of interest that are identified are thoroughly vetted by EOCME for fair balance, scientific objectivity, and patient care recommendations. EOCME is committed to providing its learners with CME activities that promote improvements or quality in healthcare and not a specific proprietary business or a commercial interest.

The planning committee, staff, authors, and editors listed below have identified no financial relationships or relationships to products or devices they or their spouse/life partner have with commercial interest related to the content of this CME activity:

Bianca Bae, MPAP, PA-C; Janelle Brown, MPAS, PA-C; Toni Beth Jackson, MMS, PA-C; Pradeep Kutty-sankaran; Lynne Meccariello, PA-C, MPAS; Aimee Salzer Pragle, DMSc, MMSc, MSPH, PA-C; Melissa Rodriguez, DMSc, PA-C, FAAPA, FAPAOG; Jenna Rolfs, DMSc, PA-C; Christina Saldanha, PA-C, NCMP; Elijah A.J. Salzer, DMSc, PA-C, NYSAFE, C-EFM; Melissa Shaffron, MPAS, PA-C; Ami Robinson Steele, DMSc, PA-C, DFAAPA; Doreen Thomas-Payne, MSN, BSN, RN, PMHNP-BC; Elyse Watkins, DHSc, PA-C, DFAAPA, NCMP; Kimberly Weikel, MPAS, PA-C

UNAPPROVED/OFF-LABEL USE DISCLOSURE

The EOCME requires CME faculty to disclose to the participants:

1. When products or procedures being discussed are off-label, unlabelled, experimental, and/or investigational (not US Food and Drug Administration [FDA] approved); and
2. Any limitations on the information presented, such as data that are preliminary or that represent ongoing research, interim analyses, and/or unsupported opinions. Faculty may discuss information about pharmaceutical agents that is outside of FDA-approved labelling. This information is intended solely for CME and is not intended to promote off-label use of these medications. If you have any questions, contact the medical affairs department of the manufacturer for the most recent prescribing information.

TO ENROLL

The CME program is available to all *Physician Assistant Clinics* subscribers at no additional fee. To subscribe to the *Physician Assistant Clinics*, call customer service at 1-800-654-2452 or sign up online at www.physicianassistant.theclinics.com.

METHOD OF PARTICIPATION

In order to claim credit, participants must complete the following:

1. Complete enrolment as indicated above
2. Read the activity
3. Complete the CME Test and Evaluation. Participants must achieve a score of 70% on the test. All CME Tests and Evaluations must be completed online

CME INQUIRIES/SPECIAL NEEDS

For all CME inquiries or special needs, please contact elsevierCME@elsevier.com.

Contributors

CONSULTING EDITORS

KIM ZUBER, PAC, MS
American Academy of Nephrology PAs, St Petersburg, Florida

JANE S. DAVIS, DNP
Division of Nephrology, University of Alabama at Birmingham, Birmingham, Alabama

EDITOR

ELYSE WATKINS, DHSc, PA-C, DFAAPA, NCMP
Associate Professor, University of Lynchburg School of PA Medicine, Doctor of Medical Science Program, Lynchburg, Virginia; Assistant Professor, Florida State University School of PA Practice, Tallahassee, Florida

AUTHORS

BIANCA BAE, MPAP, PA-C
Kindbody, Los Angeles, California

JANELLE BROWN, MPAS, PA-C
Ob/Gyn Physician Assistant, Baylor Scott and White Healthcare, Lakeway, Texas

TONI BETH JACKSON, MMS, PA-C
Assistant Professor, Wake Forest University School of Medicine, Department of PA Studies, Winston-Salem, North Carolina

LYNNE MECCARIELLO, PA-C, MPAS
Department of Quality and Patient Safety, NewYork-Presbyterian, New York, New York

AIMEE SALZER PRAGLE, DMSc, MMSc, MSPH, PA-C
Physician Assistant, University of Florida Health–Family Medicine, Jacksonville, Florida

MELISSA RODRIGUEZ, DMSc, PA-C, FAAPA
OBGYN PA, Department of Obstetrics and Gynecology, AdventHealth Central Florida South Division, Orlando, Florida

JENNA ROLFS, DMSc, PA-C
Assistant Professor, PA Medicine Program Director, University of Lynchburg, Lynchburg, Virginia

CHRISTINA SALDANHA, PA-C, NCMP
PA, Winston-Salem, North Carolina

ELIJAH A.J. SALZER, DMSc, PA-C, NYSAFE, C-EFM
Clinical Professor, Department of Physician Assistant Studies, Pace University-Lenox Hill Hospital, New York, New York; Staff Physician Assistant in Gynecology, Eastchester Medical Associates, P.C., Bronx, New York

MELISSA SHAFFRON, DMSc, MPAS, PA-C
Associate Program Director/Director of Clinical Education, School of PA Medicine, University of Lynchburg, Lynchburg, Virginia

AMI ROBINSON STEELE, DMSc, PA-C, DFAAPA
Physician Assistant, Doctor of Medical Science, Distinguished Fellow of the American Academy of Physician Assistants, Associate Professor and Director Department of Physician Assistant Studies, College of Health Sciences, Gardner-Webb University, Boiling Springs, North Carolina

ELYSE WATKINS, DHSc, PA-C, DFAAPA, NCMP
Associate Professor, University of Lynchburg School of PA Medicine, Doctor of Medical Science Program, Lynchburg, Virginia; Assistant Professor, Florida State University School of PA Practice, Tallahassee, Florida

KIMBERLY WEIKEL, MPAS, PA-C
Ob/Gyn Physician Assistant, Instructor, Department of Obstetrics and Gynecology, University of Colorado Anschutz Medical Campus, Aurora, Colorado

Contents

Aimee Salzer Pragle

> This article discusses several areas regarding women and heart disease to provide a further understanding of this disease and the importance of improved care for women. The history of heart disease in women is explored in this article to provide a foundation for understanding the beginnings of this disease and the perceptions our society has regarding how heart disease affects women. A discussion of preventative risk strategies and treatments available guides clinicians in prevention and treatment. Despite advances, continued focus on this topic is needed for improving the heart health of women.

Jenna Rolfs

> Infectious processes in the obstetric and gynecologic patient are common and require a thorough understanding of the disease state to ensure appropriate treatment and follow-up. In the obstetric patient, infectious processes are important to identify early to avoid risks of preterm labor, low birth weight, pyelonephritis, or preeclampsia. In the gynecologic patient, complications can arise if infections are left untreated. This article discusses the most common infectious diseases encountered in both obstetric and gynecologic patients.

Ami Robinson Steele and Elyse Watkins

> Because more than 200,000 women patients are diagnosed annually, health-care providers must be equipped to care for patients at risk for breast cancer and those diagnosed with or facing treatment of the disease. With so many types of breast cancer, the presentation and treatment options vary based on the molecular profile, cancer staging, and patient preference. Many patients undergo months or years of treatment, often suffering significant side effects. Survivorship begins at diagnosis, journeys through treatment, and continues throughout the patient's life. Understanding the provider's role in screening, diagnosis, treatment, and survivorship enables PAs to offer evidence-based, compassionate care for patients with breast cancer and survivors.

This article seeks to educate providers on the prevalence, pathogenesis, evaluation, management, and treatment of common causes of nonobstetric gynecologic pelvic pain. Causes of pelvic pain discussed in detail include primary dysmenorrhea, endometriosis, pelvic inflammatory disease, functional ovarian cysts, ovarian torsion, leiomyomas, and adenomyosis. After reading, providers should have a better understanding of how to approach a patient presenting with pelvic pain.

Behavioral health disorders commonly present in obstetrics and gynecology. These diagnoses can be directly correlated to changes in reproductive stages, such as adolescence and pregnancy. During these transitions patients are at risk for new diagnosis or exacerbation of symptoms. As such, utilization of screening tools and understanding of patient presentation is imperative. Delay of treatment can negatively impact quality of life for the patient and during pregnancy, led to poor fetal outcomes. This article focuses on the common mood disorders treated in obstetrics and gynecology, including depression, anxiety, postpartum depression, and premenstrual syndrome. Each is discussed as it relates to reproductive lifespan changes and the DSM-5 criteria for diagnosis. Considerations for treatment secondary to pregnancy, lactation, and side effects are also reviewed.

Fragmentation of care between primary care providers and specialists contributes to delayed infertility diagnoses and treatment. Women's health physician assistants (PAs) have the unique opportunity to provide noninvasive yet effective fertility treatments for patients with ovulatory dysfunction. Primary women's health providers doing ovulation induction have become more common; however, the lack of knowledge and experience can limit PAs from providing this service. Although reproductive endocrinology and infertility specialists have traditionally provided these services, PAs can be effective in managing these patients with the appropriate training and knowledge.

Pelvic organ prolapse (POP) is a very common condition that effects many women, increasing incidence with each decade of life particularly for women who have had at least one vaginal delivery. Other risk factors include connective tissue disorders such as Ehlers–Danlos syndrome, obesity, and genetics. POP is a clinical diagnosis and can oftentimes be diagnosed on history alone because patients will describe the sensation of a bulge in the vagina. Treatments range from expectant management, pessaries, physical therapy, and surgery, with pessaries being the first-line treatment.

Toni Beth Jackson

Pregnancy loss is a common outcome of pregnancy with loss in the first trimester being most common. Although specific risk factors exist for early, late, and recurrent pregnancy loss, they share many of the same risk factors. Providers must be aware of the appropriate approach and specific management of a patient experiencing a loss at any stage of pregnancy.

Kimberly Weikel and Elyse Watkins

This article provides an overview of gestational trophoblastic disease and gestational trophoblastic neoplasia, two conditions resulting from aberrant fertilization. After reading, providers should be able to promptly initiate an appropriate work-up and formulate a diagnosis in anticipation of managing or referring to gynecologic oncology. The current recommendations regarding patient education and surveillance are also discussed.

Lynne Meccariello

Gestational diabetes mellitus (GDM) is the most common medical complication of pregnancy, affecting approximately 7% of pregnancies in the United States. Increasing obesity rates as well as insulin resistance are contributing factors to both type II DM and GDM. Proper screening and treatment are key in minimizing complications to both mother and fetus. Maternal risks include preeclampsia, shoulder dystocia, and increased risk of operative delivery. Fetal risks include neonatal hypoglycemia, brachial plexus injury, and jaundice. Long-term sequelae include progression to type II diabetes for both mother and infant. Timeliness of screening and treatment are the keys to minimizing maternal and neonatal complications.

Elijah A.J. Salzer

Hypertensive disorders of pregnancy complicate up to 10% of all pregnancies and cause approximately 16% of all maternal deaths. These entities have increased significantly in the past 25 years and are disproportionately seen in Black patients. Individuals with a history of preeclampsia are at high risk of cardiovascular disease later in life, particularly those patients who developed early-onset preeclampsia (occurring before 34 weeks gestational age). Although all patients with these disorders have hypertension, the preeclamptic syndromes are distinct from gestational hypertension and chronic hypertension because they may involve the renal, hepatic, hematologic, pulmonary, and/or central nervous systems.

PHYSICIAN ASSISTANT CLINICS

SERIES OF RELATED INTEREST

Medical Clinics
https://www.medical.theclinics.com/

THE CLINICS ARE AVAILABLE ONLINE!
Access your subscription at:
www.theclinics.com

FORTHCOMING ISSUES

October 2022
Nutrition in Patient Care
Scott W.H. Keller

January 2023
Emergency Medicine
Dan Tzizik, Editor

April 2023
Pharmacology
Rebecca Maxson, Editor

RECENT ISSUES

April 2022
The Kidney
Kim Zuber and Jane Davis, Editors

January 2022
Preventive Medicine
Stephanie Neary, Editor

October 2021
Gastroenterology
Jennifer R. Eames, Editor

SERIES OF RELATED INTEREST

Medical Clinics
https://www.medical.theclinics.com

THE CLINICS ARE AVAILABLE ONLINE!
Access your subscription at:
www.theclinics.com

Foreword

It's a Woman's World

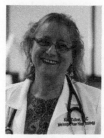 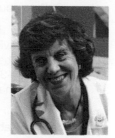

Kim Zuber, PAC, MS   Jane S. Davis, DNP
Consulting Editors

One of the earliest breakthroughs in women's health occurred in 1850 when Dr Ignaz Semmelweis discovered that cleanliness did indeed count.[1] After observing the incidence of childbirth fever at physician deliveries was 10 to 20 times greater that of midwife deliveries, he proposed that physicians, by not washing hands between patients, were responsible.

Care of women has traditionally been relegated to second place in medicine. A prime example is heart disease trials with only male subjects. This issue of *Physician Assistant Clinics* gives women's health and its practitioners the stature they deserve. Authored by caring, knowledgeable practitioners, it is a fascinating look at an area often undervalued in medical education. Edited by Elyse Watkins, an experienced obstetrics and gynecology (Ob/Gyn) physician assistant, this issue provides 13 informative articles that look at women's health. These run the gamut from Ob/Gyn to heart disease to cancer to women's mental health. It is a wonderful asset for everyone, even those not practicing Ob/Gyn.

We would like to take this opportunity to introduce ourselves. After having been guest editors for 5 issues of *Physician Assistant Clinics*, we have taken on the position of executive editors. We owe a debt of gratitude to Jim Van Rhee, who was the original executive editor and has held that position since the journal's inception in 2016. We

Physician Assist Clin 7 (2022) xiii–xiv
https://doi.org/10.1016/j.cpha.2022.03.006
2405-7991/22/© 2022 Published by Elsevier Inc.

physicianassistant.theclinics.com

look forward to making Jim proud and getting to read all these wonderful articles from our brilliant and caring colleagues.

Kim Zuber, PAC, MS
American Academy of Nephrology PAs
131 31st Avenue North
St Petersburg, FL 33704, USA

Jane S. Davis, DNP
Division of Nephrology
University of Alabama at Birmingham
3605 Oakdale Road
Birmingham, AL 35223, USA

E-mail addresses:
zuberkim@yahoo.com (K. Zuber)
jsdavis@uabmc.edu (J.S. Davis)

REFERENCE

1. Markel H. PBS Newshour. 2015. Available at: https://www.pbs.org/newshour/health/ignaz-semmelweis-doctor-prescribed-hand-washing. Accessed March 24, 2022.

Preface

Why Obstetrics and Gynecology?

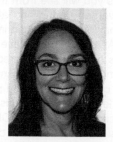

Elyse Watkins, DHSc, PA-C, DFAAPA, NCMP
Editor

Over two decades ago, two physicians, recently out of residency, took a chance and hired their first physician assistant (PA) to work in their obstetrics and gynecology (Ob/Gyn) practice. I was not only their first PA, I was also the first PA in the county whose population was larger than that of the states of Wyoming, North Dakota, South Dakota, Alaska, and Vermont. I remember fighting with the labor and delivery nurses to take my orders for even the most basic of tasks. In addition, I educated other ob/gyn physicians on how to utilize PAs in their practice. I knew I had been successful when labor and delivery nurses from several hospitals came to see me as patients. I started precepting PA students, and although most did not love the specialty nearly as much as me, I enjoyed showing them exactly how a PA can function in a busy Ob/Gyn practice.

Since that time, the number of PAs working in Ob/Gyn across the United States has increased, albeit much slower than in other specialties. According to the National Commission on Certification of PAs, only 1.2% of certified PAs practice in Ob/Gyn settings.[1] While the total number of PAs in Ob/Gyn has increased 11.4% since 2016, the percentage of PAs working in this speciality has not changed. Many PA students who want to work in Ob/Gyn have had to take jobs in family medicine and create niches where they can practice primary care gynecology. All the while, their hearts are still in the specialty practice. I know that each one of them would jump at the chance to work in an Ob/Gyn practice if given the opportunity. Because of various barriers that persist, we are still vastly underrepresented in this specialty.

The authors who have collaborated and written articles for this issue work in a myriad of settings, including reproductive endocrinology and infertility, general Ob/Gyn, family medicine, and labor and delivery. Some are also teaching in PA programs, chairing PA programs, first assisting in the operating room, creating their own practices, and seeking additional credentials to enhance their ability to care for women during and after their reproductive years. Some of these authors have personal experience with the disease states they describe. Whether or not they have personal experience, all have

Physician Assist Clin 7 (2022) xv–xvi
https://doi.org/10.1016/j.cpha.2022.03.005
2405-7991/22/© 2022 Published by Elsevier Inc.

cared for patients who were at their most vulnerable. Despite the origin of their perspective, their love of caring for women is clear.

It is for these reasons I was delighted to help create an issue on Ob/Gyn topics written by PAs who can use their expertise and experience not only to disseminate clinical information but also to encourage other PAs and PA students who are thinking about transitioning into Ob/Gyn or one of its subspecialties. As you will see from the article titles, we cover various topics relevant to caring for women during and after their reproductive years, including cardiovascular health, behavioral health, and infectious diseases commonly encountered in clinical practice. All publications have content limits, which meant many important and timely topics had to be deferred. These include lesbian care, transgender health, sexual health, menopause, and many others. It is hoped that another group of PAs will be willing to come together and join on a future issue where we can focus on some of these other topics. While this issue is not intended to include all relevant information in the clinical practice of Ob/Gyn, it is a representation of the talent in our profession. As such, I celebrate my collegues and all of you who are taking the time to read these articles.

Elyse Watkins, DHSc, PA-C, DFAAPA, NCMP
University of Lynchburg School of
PA Medicine
Doctor of Medical Science Program
1501 Lakeside Drive
Lynchburg, VA 24501, USA

E-mail address:
Elysewatkins.five@gmail.com

REFERENCE

1. National Commission on Certification of PAs, Inc. 2020 Statistical profile of certified PAs: an annual report of the National Commission on Certification of PAs. 2021. Available at: http://www.nccpa.net/research. Accessed April 9, 2022.

Female Heart Disease

Aimee Salzer Pragle, DMSc, MMSc, MSPH, PA-C*

KEYWORDS

- Heart disease • Women's health • Female health • Preventative medicine
- Cardiac risk factors

KEY POINTS

- Heart disease is the number one cause of death of women in the United States.
- The belief that cardiac disease is more benign in women than in men has led to less aggressive diagnosis and management of the disease in women.
- As the population of older women continues to increase, the number of patients with heart disease will continue to increase.
- Although there has been improvement with time, there continues to be more of a focus on male health in cardiac research compared with female health.
- Clinicians can play a crucial role in improving the health of their female patients by following the most recent guidelines to encourage patients in embracing healthy lifestyle choices and implementing prevention and treatment strategies.

INTRODUCTION

Heart disease is the number one cause of death of women in the United States. In 2017, 1 out of every 5 female deaths was attributed to heart disease. This totals more than 400,000 women per year dying of heart disease.[1] The perception is often that more men die of heart disease than women. However, women are almost as likely as men to die of a heart-related cause. The belief that cardiac disease is more benign in women than men has led to less aggressive diagnosis and management of the disease in female patients.[2] This unfortunately can have grave consequences, increasing the risk of morbidity and mortality in our patients.

Although men develop heart disease approximately 10 years earlier than women, as women advance in age their risk becomes comparable to men.[3] When women do develop heart disease, they typically have a worse prognosis than men once they have had a myocardial infarction (MI).[4] It is concerning that women have higher mortalities than men with heart disease. Within 1 year of an unrecognized MI, 44% of women will die compared with 27% of men.[5] In addition, within 6 years of an MI, 46% of women will develop heart failure (congestive heart failure), whereas only 22% of men will develop this condition.[6]

University of Florida Health–Family Medicine, 4322 Birmingham Road, Jacksonville, FL 32207, USA
* Corresponding author.
E-mail address: Aimee.Pragle@jax.ufl.edu

Physician Assist Clin 7 (2022) 409–418
https://doi.org/10.1016/j.cpha.2022.02.001
2405-7991/22/© 2022 Elsevier Inc. All rights reserved.

It continues to be common for heart disease to be missed and diagnosis to be delayed in women. Female patients continue to perceive breast cancer as their number one risk for death. About 56% of women identify heart disease as the number one cause of death for their gender.[7] However, only 13% identified it as the greatest risk to their health.

There have been many advances in the study and treatment of heart disease and women. Over the past 30 years, there have been significant decreases in heart disease mortality for both men and women, particularly in individuals 65 years and above. However, recent studies show that for younger women less than 55 years of age, there appears to be an increase in the incidence of heart disease compared with the past.[8] The underlying mechanisms that contribute to these findings need to be researched in more depth to identify further interventions and prevention that can reduce the risk of the development of heart disease.

As the population of older women continues to increase, the number of patients with heart disease will continue to increase. Health care providers must be given the tools necessary for helping to reduce the risk of women developing heart disease. However, continued efforts are needed to progress these efforts. A need for increased training for health care providers to recognize the symptoms of heart disease in women has been identified. In a study of medical students nationwide, it was identified that only 43% of medical students found their medical training helped to increase their knowledge of the relationship of sex and gender in the effective delivery of medical care. Only 35% of these students thought they had the necessary tools to take care of patients based on sex and gender differences.[9]

UNIQUE PRESENTATION OF HEART DISEASE IN WOMEN

The risk factors and presenting signs and symptoms women have can be vastly different compared with how men present with heart disease.[10] Researchers have shown that the presentation and contributing risk factors of heart disease in women are different from those of men. The protective benefits of estrogen that reduce with age in women are a key component for the differences in heart disease presentation.[11] The presence of estrogen helps to delay the development of elevated cholesterol in women, which reduces the risk of developing heart disease.

Women are more likely to have an atypical presentation of heart disease. Chest pain is regarded as the hallmark symptom in identifying a patient with acute coronary syndrome. However, women often do not have the cardinal symptoms that help in including cardiac issues in the differential diagnosis. Being a woman of young age and not having classic left-sided chest pain are the 2 strongest indicators that a patient with a cardiac presentation will be misdiagnosed and mistakenly discharged from the emergency department instead of being appropriately evaluated and treated.[12]

Data from the Framingham Study identified that it is more common for women to have angina pectoris than men. In contrast, men are more likely to present with MI and sudden death.[13] Clinicians should be acutely aware that any woman who presents with symptoms at all concerning for heart disease should receive a comprehensive cardiac workup. Dismissing symptoms as being psychosomatic, gastrointestinal, or musculoskeletal can cause misdiagnosis and increase morbidity and mortality of the patient as well as increase legal liability of the provider.[14]

Possible complications of pregnancy can increase the risk for heart disease. Preeclampsia, which is high blood pressure with end-organ involvement during pregnancy, is a risk factor that can increase the development of heart disease later in life. In addition, the presence of heart disease before pregnancy may increase the risk for the development of pregnancy complications.[15] Women who have a preterm delivery defined as birth at less than 37 weeks' gestation are at greater risk for cardio-vascular problems in the future. The reasons for this remain poorly understood; however, it is thought that mechanisms such as inflammation, infection, and vascular complications are related to preterm delivery in women and thus can further exacerbate underlying cardiac problems.[16]

Decreased production of estrogen and weight gain that can occur in middle age increases risk factors for heart disease for women. Premenopausal patients have protection owing to the cardioprotective properties of estrogen. However, premature menopause owing to oophorectomy or chemical ablation of the ovaries is also a risk factor, particularly if the patient does not receive adequate exogenous estrogen support. The addition of hormone replacement therapy in naturally postmenopausal patients is not a benefit long term and can increase the risk of heart disease, particularly when progestins are used.

Treatment for breast cancer can increase the risk for heart disease. There is a risk of the heart being exposed to ionizing radiation during radiotherapy for breast cancer. Patients who already have preexisting cardiac issues are at significantly greater risk of developing cardiac complications following radiotherapy.[17] Patients with breast cancer who use certain chemotherapies are at significantly increased risk of developing cardiac disease, specifically, left ventricular dysfunction and heart failure (see Ami Robinson Steele and Elyse Watkins' article, "Breast Cancer, " in this issue). It is a medical success that breast cancer treatments have helped to improve overall survival rates; however, clinicians must understand the increased cardiac risks that occur owing to these treatments and be vigilant in conducting evidence-based screening and evaluation in women who have undergone radiotherapy.

PREVENTATIVE MEASURES

More than 200 risk factors contribute to heart disease. As more research is completed, continued data on known risk factors as well as the discovery of new risk factors are identified.[18] The traditional risk factors for men are also risk factors for women. However, there are gender differences in the epidemiology of these risk factors in prevalence rates and relative risk. Major identified risk factors for developing heart disease for men and women include tobacco use, hypertension, diabetes mellitus, dyslipidemia, obesity, sedentary lifestyle, and an unhealthy diet.[19] Findings from the longitudinal, observational Nurses' Health Study have identified the vital importance of modification of lifestyles to reduce the risk of developing heart disease. It has been shown that women can reduce the risk of coronary events by more than 80% if they actively incorporate healthy lifestyle components.[20]

Some steps can be taken toward the goal of reducing risk factors. All too often, health care providers are less likely to educate female patients regarding risk factors in comparison to male patients. It is not as common for women to be provided advice about quitting smoking or to receive valuable pharmaceutical interventions, such as aspirin therapy and cholesterol-lowering medications. In addition, health care providers are less likely to refer women for diagnostic tests, such as electrocardiograms. Younger women in particular are more likely than men to receive the wrong diagnosis and to be sent home even if they are experiencing a cardiac event.[21] Working to reduce risk factors that contribute to heart disease should be the main goal of health care providers in the primary care setting.

Lifestyle plays a critical role in reducing the risk of developing heart disease in women. The Nurses' Health Study followed 84,129 women who had no comorbidities of cardiovascular disease, cancer, or diabetes. These participants were followed for

14 years.[22] Participants in the study were categorized as low risk if they did not smoke, were not overweight, had low consumption of alcohol, exercised half an hour a day, and consumed a low-fat, high-fiber diet. Women in the low-risk category were significantly less likely to develop heart disease as compared with those who were in the higher-risk category. This study demonstrates the importance of a healthy lifestyle in reducing the risk of heart disease in women.

Smoking is the cause of more deaths from heart disease and stroke than any other disease.[23] In developed countries, 24% of all male and 7% of all female deaths can be attributed to cigarette smoking.[24] Cigarette smoking increases the risk of developing heart disease in both men and women. Passive smoking exposure is also a risk. Younger patients who smoke are at higher risk of developing heart disease. For female smokers aged 18 to 49 years, their risk of having an MI was 13 times greater than for those who did not smoke. It is promising to note that once the patients quit smoking for at least a month, their risk dropped to a similar range as nonsmokers.[25] All patients who are smokers should work toward smoking cessation. Smoking cessation has been shown to effectively reduce mortality and morbidity. When an individual stops smoking, the onset of heart disease can be delayed by about 10 years.[26] Patients should be encouraged to continue to refrain if they do not smoke and to quit smoking if they have developed the unhealthy habit of smoking. Many tobacco cessation options exist but are beyond the scope of this article.

Hypertension is a major risk factor for developing heart disease. Men generally have a higher blood pressure than women. However, as women age, the prevalence and severity of hypertension increase. By age 65 years, more women than men have hypertension.[27] It is predicted that more women than men will have hypertension: by 2025, the prevalence of hypertension worldwide is expected to increase by 9% in men and 13% in women.[28] Thus, female patients should have their blood pressure checked regularly.

More than 15 million women in the United States have diabetes.[29] In women, diabetes can lead to worse outcomes than for men. Women with diabetes are twice as likely to develop heart disease. In addition, they are more likely to have an MI at an earlier age and more likely for it to be fatal.[30] One of the reasons for women to have greater morbidity and mortality with diabetes and heart disease is that they are treated less acutely than men. Within 1 year of a diabetes diagnosis, women were less likely to be prescribed cholesterol medication and heart-protective medication.[31] Another concerning factor is that women are more likely to be obese at the time of diabetes diagnosis, which further increases the risk of heart disease. There are evidence-based recommendations for routine evaluations by primary care providers, including checking blood glucose and hemoglobin A_{1c} for preventative screening. The American Diabetes Association recommends that women 45 years and older have a fasting glucose completed every 3 years for screening.[32]

Dyslipidemia is the most prevalent risk factor for heart disease with approximately 47.1% of women having this condition.[33] Dyslipidemia typically does not become a major risk for women until they have entered menopause. Lifestyle modifications with a focus on diet and exercise can greatly reduce the risk of developing high cholesterol. Guidelines from the American Heart Association and American College of Cardiology recommend that statins should be prescribed for patients who are moderate or high risk.[34] Despite these recommendations, women who meet the criteria are less likely to be prescribed statins than men.[35]

Obesity, particularly visceral adiposity, increases the risk of developing heart disease. In the United States, more than 2 in 3 adults are overweight or obese, and the prevalence of obesity is greater among women.[36] The Framingham Heart Study identified that obesity increases the risk of developing coronary artery disease by 64% in women, and only by 46% in men.[37] Despite the significant impact of obesity on their health, more than 25% of women state they do not engage in exercise regularly.

An emphasis on preventative medicine and reducing the risk of developing heart disease is crucial for addressing the needs of women and their cardiac health. Medical providers can carefully review medical history and laboratory results to identify the appropriate pharmaceutical interventions and health education strategies to provide patients with the tools needed to reduce their cardiac risks.

TREATMENT GOALS

Despite advances in recognizing gender differences in heart disease, women continue to have a higher rate of MI complications, such as heart rupture, cardiogenic shock, and atrial fibrillation, than men.[38] Within the first year of their first MI, 38% of women die compared with 25% of men.[39] To reduce these disparities, continued focus on evidence-based treatment strategies needs to be a primary goal of clinicians.

In 2007, the American Heart Association published a document focused on evidence-based guidelines to prevent heart disease in women. For the first time, recommendations for early screening and conducting a complete risk assessment were made.[40] The guidelines were updated in 2019.

Regardless of risk category, a heart-healthy diet is recommended for all patients for optimal cardiac health. A diet rich in fish should be consumed at least twice a week and fruits, vegetables and whole grains consumed on a regular basis. The diet should be limited in saturated fats, sugar, alcohol, and sodium. Complete avoidance of trans fats is recommended. In addition, women should exercise for a minimum of 150 minutes per week at a moderate-intensity exercise, such as brisk walking.[41]

Patients who are considered at risk for developing heart disease have one or more of the following major risk factors: cigarette smoking, obesity, physical inactivity, family history of coronary artery disease, hypertension, or dyslipidemia. Women with other conditions, such as subclinical vascular disease; metabolic syndrome; autoimmune vascular disease, such as lupus; history of preeclampsia; gestational diabetes; and pregnancy-induced hypertension, are also at risk. Lifestyle changes are recommended for those who are considered at risk as well as pharmaceutical interventions as necessary. Statins should be considered in patients with elevated cholesterol. All patients should obtain the goal of optimal blood pressure. Joint national commission (JNC). Guidelines recommend initiation of pharmacologic treatment when blood pressure is 150/90 mm Hg or higher in adults 60 years and older or 140/90 mm Hg or higher in adults younger than 60 years. In patients with hypertension and diabetes, initiation of pharmacologic treatment is recommended if blood pressure is 140/90 mm Hg or higher regardless of age.[42] In addition, it is recommended for an A_{1C} less than 7% to reduce cardiac risk.[43]

Aspirin has been shown to be effective in secondary prevention of heart disease for both men and women. The Women's Health Study evaluated more than 40,000 women who were greater than 45 years. The women in this study were assigned to either receive a low dose of aspirin every day or a placebo for 10 years.[44] Results of the study showed there was a significant benefit for women who took low-dose aspirin vs placebo in reducing the risk of developing heart disease or stroke. Although aspirin is beneficial, there is some risk of bleeding with this medication. Thus, it is only recommended for patients who meet high-risk criteria for heart disease or do not have contraindications.

Statin therapy is an effective medication to aid in the prevention of heart disease. New guidelines for the use of statin therapy were provided in 2013 by the American College of Cardiology and the American Heart Association. These guidelines stated that statins should be prescribed in all patients with heart disease who meet criteria, as well as asymptomatic adults aged 40 to 75 years without a history of heart disease who have (1) low-density lipoprotein (LDL) cholesterol level greater than 189; (2) LDL cholesterol level of 70 to 189.[45]

Angiotensin II receptor blockers are recommended for women after they have sustained an MI or if they have heart failure. Beta-blockers and aldosterone blockade are recommended in some patients, if necessary, after they have had an MI. Patients who have developed heart failure or a heart arrhythmia benefit from the addition of these medications.[46]

Other interventions that are popular offer no benefit and may even be harmful for use. These include antioxidant supplements, such as vitamin E, C, and beta-carotene for primary or secondary prevention. There is no need for folic acid replacement for use in the treatment or prevention of heart disease. In addition, postmenopausal hormone replacement therapy is not indicated for the use of heart disease prevention. There is research supporting the benefits of CoQ10 supplementation for cardiac health. Doses of 200 mg/d or higher are safe and contribute to reducing oxidative stress, decreasing vascular stiffness, and improving endothelial function.[47] Omega 3 fatty acids have also shown cardioprotective benefits for patients.[48]

BARRIERS AND CHALLENGES

Women can present with symptoms more atypically than men and are less likely to experience classic symptoms, such as left-sided anterior chest pain. They are more likely to experience atypical symptoms, such as back or stomach pain, chest pressure or tightness, dizziness, fatigue, indigestion, nausea, or shortness of breath. Women may experience prodromal symptoms up to a year before they experience an MI. These symptoms may include sleep disturbances, weakness, anxiety, and unusual tiredness. Often clinicians will attribute these symptoms to depression and anxiety and not recognize the need to do a workup for cardiac disease.

Some women with heart disease may not even have any symptoms. Silent heart disease is not diagnosed until the disease progresses and the risk of developing MIs, arrhythmias, or heart failure is elevated.[49]

Routine diagnostic tools available for the evaluation of cardiac symptoms do not always provide the same sensitivity and specificity for women. For example, the exercise treadmill, which is used for evaluation of ischemia, has less ability to detect abnormalities in female patients.[50]

Further barriers exist for women of color, particularly black women with heart disease. There is a 69% higher death rate from heart disease for black women compared with non-Hispanic whites. They are also more likely to experience bias in the health care system.[51]

SUMMARY

This article has provided a review of heart disease and its impact on the health of women. Throughout history, there have been immense challenges and barriers reducing the optimal care women receive for their heart health. Although there has been a positive focus on improving cardiac health for women, female patients continue to be more likely to die of heart disease than any other disease. Identifying risk and preventing disease through evidence-based intervention is the cornerstone of care for reducing the morbidity and mortality caused by this disease.

Clinicians can play a crucial role in improving the health of their female patients by following the most recent guidelines to encourage patients in embracing healthy lifestyle choices and implementing prevention and treatment strategies. Educating women to recognize the signs and symptoms of heart disease empowers them to have a better understanding of their health and know how to respond if a health event occurs.

CLINICS CARE POINTS

- Healthy lifestyle coaching should be provided to patients, as it can reduce the risk of coronary artery disease in women by more than 80%.
- Female patients should have their blood pressure checked regularly as hypertension is a major risk factor for developing heart disease.
- The American Diabetes Association recommends that women 45 years and older have a fasting glucose completed every 3 years for screening.
- Women who meet high-risk criteria for heart disease should recieve a low dose of aspirin every day to reduce risk of heart disease.

DISCLOSURE

No disclosures to make.

REFERENCES

1. Centers for Disease Control and Prevention, National Center for Health Statistics. Underlying Cause of Death 1999–2017 on CDC WONDER Online Database, released December 2018. Data are from the Multiple Cause of Death Files, 1999–2017, as compiled from data provided by the 57 vital statistics jurisdictions through the Vital Statistics Cooperative Program. Available at: https://wonder.cdc.gov/wonder. Accessed June 7, 2001.
2. Garcia M, Mulvagh S, Merz N, et al. Cardiovascular disease in women: clinical perspectives. Circ Res 2016;118(8):1273–93.
3. Humphries K, Izadnegadar M, Sedlak T, et al. Sex differences in cardiovascular disease – impact on care and outcomes. Front Neuroendocrinol 2017;46:46–70.
4. Appelman Y, Van Rijn BB, Ten Haaf M, et al. Sex differences in cardiovascular risk factors and disease prevention. Atherosclerosis 2015;241:211–8.
5. Pathak L, Shirodkar S, Ruparelia R, et al. Coronary artery disease in women. Indian Heart J 2017;69(4):532–8.
6. Virani S, Alonso A, Aparicio H, et al. Heart disease and stroke statistics – 2021 update: a report from the American Heart Association. Circulation 2021;143:254–743.
7. Mosca L, Hammond G, Mochari-Greenberger H, et al. Fifteen-year trends in awareness of heart disease in women: results of the 2012 American Heart Association National Survey. Circulation 2013;127(11):1254–63, e 1 – 29.
8. Wilmot KA, O'Flaherty M, Capewell S, et al. Coronary heart disease mortality declines in the United States from 1979 through 2011: evidence for stagnation in young adults, especially women. Circulation 2015;132:997–1002.

9. Jenkins MR, Hermann A, Tashijian A, et al. Sex and gender in medical education: a national student survey. Biol Sex Differ 2016;7(Suppl 1):45.

10. Zhao M, Vaartjes I, Graham D, et al. Sex differences in risk factor management of coronary heart disease across three regions. Heart 2017;103:1587–94.

11. Brush JE, Krumholz HM, Greene EJ, et al. Sex differences in symptom phenotypes among patients with acute myocardial infarction. Circulation 2020; 13(2):13–6.

12. Andersson C, Ramachandran S. Epidemiology of cardiovascular disease in young individuals. Nat Rev Cardiol 2018;(15):230–40.

13. Fabian S, Perez-Quillis C, Leischik R, et al. Epidemiology of coronary heart disease and acute coronary syndrome. Ann Transl Med 2016;4(13):256.

14. Walsh M, Greenberger P, Campbell S, et al. Knowledge, attitudes and beliefs regarding cardiovascular disease in women: the Women's Heart Alliance. J Am Coll Cardiol 2017;70(2):123–32.

15. Milner KA, Funk M, Arnold A. Typical symptoms are predictive of acute coronary syndromes in women. Am Heart J 2002;143:283–8.

16. Listen to your heart: women and heart disease. National Heart, Lung and Blood Institute. Available at: https://www.nhibi.nih.gov/healthtopics/eduation-and-awareness/heart-truth/listen-to-your-heart. Accessed June 11, 2021.

17. Kessous R, Shoham-Vardi I, Parinete G, et al. An association between preterm delivery and long-term maternal cardiovascular morbidity. Am J Obstet Gynecol 2013;209:368.

18. Darby SC, Ewertz M, McGale P, et al. Risk of ischemic heart disease in women after radiotherapy for breast cancer. N Engl J Med 2013;368:987–98.

19. Mehta P, Wei J, Wenger N. Ischemic heart disease in women: a focus on risk factors. Trends Cardiovasc Med 2015;25(2):140–51.

20. LaMonte J. Physical activity, fitness, and coronary heart disease. Cardiorespiratory Fitness Cardiometabolic Dis 2019;17:295–318.

21. Hu FB, Stampfer MJ, Manson JE. Trends in the incidence of coronary heart disease and changes in diet and lifestyle in women. N Engl J Med 2000;343:530–7.

22. Harvard Health. The heart attack gender gap. 2016. Available at: https://www.health.harvard.edu/heart-health/. Accessed May 8, 2021.

23. Stampfer MJ, Hu FB, Manson JE, et al. Primary prevention of coronary heart disease in women through diet and lifestyle. N Engl J Med 2000;346:16–22.

24. Prabhat J. The hazards of smoking and the benefits of cessation: a critical summation of the epidemiological evidence in high-income countries. Epidemiol Glob Health 2020;9:e49979.

25. Gavidia M. Smoking cessation found to lower risk of cardiovascular disease. Am J Manag Care 2019;1.

26. Palmer J, Lloyd A, Lloyd S, et al. Differential risk of ST-segment elevation myocardial infarction in male and female smokers. J Am Coll Cardiol 2019;73(25): 3259–66.

27. Feeman WE. The role of cigarette smoking in atherosclerotic disease: an epidemiologic analysis. J Cardiovasc Risk 1999;6:333–6.

28. Roger VL, Go AS, Lloyd-Jones DM, et al. Heart disease and stroke statistics – 2011 update. A report from the American Heart Association. Circulation 2011; 123:18–209.

29. National Diabetes Statistics Report 2020. Estimates of diabetes and its burden in the United States. Cdc.gov/diabetes/pdfs/data/statistics/national-daibetes-statistics.

30. Kearney PM, Whelton M, Reynolds K. Global burden of hypertension: analysis of worldwide data. Lancet 2005;365:217–23.
31. American Diabetes Association. Cardiovascular disease and risk management: standards of medical care in diabetes – 2019. Diabetes Care 2019;(42):103–23.
32. Koerbel G, Korytkowski M. Coronary heart disease in women with diabetes. Diabetes Spectr 2003;16(3):148–53.
33. Howard BV, Cowan L, Go O, et al. Adverse effects of diabetes on multiple cardiovascular risk factors in women: the Strong Heart Study. Diabetes Care 1998;21:1258–65.
34. Arnett D, Blumenthal R, Albert M, et al. 2019 ACC/AHA Guideline on the primary prevention of cardiovascular disease: a report of the American College of Cardiology/American Heart Association task force on clinical practice guidelines. J Am Coll Cardiol 2019;140(11):177–232.
35. Yusuf S, Hawken S, Ounpuu S, et al. Effect of potentially modifiable risk factors associated with myocardial infarction in 52 countries (the Interheart Study): case-control study. Lancet 2004;364:937–52.
36. Virani SS, Woodard LD, Ramsey DJ. Gender disparities in evidence-based statin therapy in patients with cardiovascular disease. Am J Cardiol 2015;115:21–6.
37. Flegal KM, Carroll MD, Kit BK, et al. Prevalence of obesity and trends in the distribution of body mass index among US adults, 1999 – 2010. JAMA 2012;307:491–7.
38. Wilson PW, Kannel WB, Silbershatz H, et al. Clustering of metabolic factors and coronary heart disease. Arch Intern Med 1999;159:1104–9.
39. Rollini F, Mfeukeu L, Modena M, et al. Assessing coronary heart disease in women. Maturitas 2009;62(3):243–7.
40. Bhupathy P, Haines C, Leinwand L. Influence of sex hormones and phytoestrogens on heart disease in men and women. Womens Health (Lond) 2010;6(1):77–95.
41. Mosca L, Benjamin EJ, Berra K. Effectiveness-based guidelines for the prevention of cardiovascular disease in women – 2011 update: a guideline from the American Heart Association. Circulation 2011;123:1243–62.
42. James P, Oparil S, Carter B. 2014 Evidence-based guideline for the management of high blood pressure in adults. JAMA 2014;311(5):507–20.
43. US Department of Health & Human Services. Physical activity guidelines for Americans. 2008. Available at: http://www.health.gov/paguidelines. Accessed March 16, 2021.
44. Ridker PM, Cook NR, Lee IM, et al. A randomized trial of low-dose aspirin in primary prevention of cardiovascular disease in women. N Engl J Med 2005;352:1293–304.
45. Stone N, Robinson J, Lichtenstein A, et al. 2013 ACC/AHA Guideline on the treatment of blood cholesterol to reduce atherosclerotic cardiovascular risk in adults. Circulation 2013;129(25).
46. Sim HW, Zheng A, Richards M. Beta-blockers and renin-angiotensin system inhibitors in acute myocardial infarction managed with in hospital coronary revascularization. Sci Rep 2020;10(1):15184.
47. Rabanal-Ruiz Y, Llanos-Gonzalez E, Alcain F. The use of coenzyme Q10 in cardiovascular disease. Antioxidants 2021;10(5):755.
48. Desnoyers M, Gilbert K, Rousseau G. Cardioprotective effects of omega-3 polyunsaturated fatty acids: dichotomy between experimental and clinical studies. Mar Drugs 2018;16(7):234.

49. Mechanic O, Grossman SA. Acute myocardial infarction. Treasure Island, Florida: StatPearls. StatPearls Publishing; 2020.
50. Vilcant V, Zeltser R. Treadmill stress testing. Treasure Island, Florida: StatPearls. StatPearls Publishing; 2021.
51. Breathett K. Latest evidence on racial inequalities and biases in advanced health care. 2020. American College of Cardiology Expert Analysis. Available at: https://www.acc.org/latest-in-cardiology/articles/2020/10/01/11/39/latest-evidence-on-racial-inequities-and-biases-in-advanced-hf. Accessed May 5, 2021.

Common Infections Encountered in Obstetrics/ Gynecology

Jenna Rolfs, DMSc, PA-C

KEYWORDS

• Bacteriuria • Cystitis • Pyelonephritis • Vaginitis • Group B streptococcus

KEY POINTS

- Untreated common infections in the obstetric/gynecologic (OB/GYN) patient can lead to preterm birth, low birth weight, pyelonephritis, and/or preeclampsia.
- Consider local antibiotic resistance patterns when prescribing empiric antibiotic therapy in the OB/GYN population.
- Universal prenatal screening is key to effective prevention of group B streptococcus.
- Avoid alcohol consumption and breastfeeding when taking metronidazole to treat common infections in the OB/GYN patient.

ASYMPTOMATIC BACTERIURIA

Asymptomatic bacteriuria is the presence of bacteria in the urine in a patient who does not exhibit any signs/symptoms of infection.[1,2] Per the US Preventative Task Force, the importance of screening for asymptomatic bacteriuria in pregnant women is because of the risks of untreated bacteriuria, which in pregnancy includes preterm labor, low birth weight, pyelonephritis, and preeclampsia.

PATHOPHYSIOLOGY/CAUSE

The prevalence of asymptomatic bacteriuria is the same between nonpregnant and pregnant patients.[1] At least one pathogen must be present in the urine to have bacteriuria, and *Escherichia coli* is the most common pathogen. However, asymptomatic bacteriuria can be polymicrobial. The prevalence of asymptomatic bacteriuria is more common in the first trimester of pregnancy.

RISK FACTORS

Common risk factors associated with asymptomatic bacteriuria include history of prior urinary tract infection (UTI), preexisting diabetes mellitus, pregnancy, older age, spinal cord injury, and long-term catheter use.[1]

The author has no commercial or financial conflicts of interest to disclose.
University of Lynchburg, 1501 Lakeside Drive, Lynchburg, VA 24501, USA
E-mail address: rolfs_je@lynchburg.edu

CLINICAL PRESENTATIONS

The clinical presentation of asymptomatic bacteriuria is primarily the absence of signs/symptoms related to a UTI, which would be dysuria, urgency, frequency, hematuria, or pubic pain.[1]

DIAGNOSIS

The diagnosis of asymptomatic bacteriuria can be made with a urine culture.[1] To diagnosis asymptomatic bacteriuria, the urine culture must show $\geq 10^5$ colony-forming units (CFU) on 2 consecutive specimens. The urine culture is obtained with a clean-catch midstream urine sample.

TREATMENT

There is no clinical indication to treat asymptomatic bacteriuria in nonpregnant patients, and some data suggest that treatment of asymptomatic bacteriuria in nonpregnant patients can contribute to antibiotic resistance.[1,3] Because of the risk factors associated with untreated asymptomatic bacteriuria in pregnancy, as well as the risk of developing pyelonephritis if left untreated, asymptomatic bacteriuria is treated in pregnancy. Appropriate antibiotic therapy regimens include the following:

- Amoxicillin 250 mg by mouth 3 times a day for 3 or 7 days
  - Alternative regimen is Amoxicillin 3 g by mouth × 1
- Cephalexin 2 or 3 g by mouth × 1
- Nitrofurantoin 200 mg by mouth × 1
  - Alternative regimen is Nitrofurantoin 100 mg by mouth 4 times a day × 3 or 7 days; an appropriate antibiotic therapy is nitrofurantoin monohydrate 100 mg by mouth 2 times a day × 7 days. Antibiotic therapy might need to be modified depending on urine culture results.

KEY POINTS

- Recurrent bacteriuria is more common in pregnant patients.[1,4]
- Asymptomatic bacteriuria should only be treated in pregnant patients.
- Asymptomatic bacteriuria in the nonpregnant women does not need to be treated.
- Screening for asymptomatic bacteriuria in pregnant women usually occurs at the first prenatal visit.
- Untreated bacteriuria can lead to preterm birth, low birth weight, pyelonephritis, preeclampsia.

URINARY TRACT INFECTIONS: ACUTE CYSTITIS

UTIs can be classified as lower UTIs, known as acute cystitis, or upper UTIs, known as pyelonephritis.[5] The most common gram-negative bacterium associated with both lower and upper UTIs is E coli. UTIs are more common in women secondary to the anatomic makeup of the female genitalia.

PATHOPHYSIOLOGY/CAUSE

Acute cystitis is classified as a lower UTI.[5] E coli, a gram-negative bacteriumum, is the most common pathogen associated with acute cystitis. Other organisms include Klebsiella, Enterobacter species, Proteus, and gram-positive organisms.

RISK FACTORS

Common risk factors associated with acute cystitis include immunosuppression, recent urinary tract instrumentation, recent antibiotic use, and advanced age.[5]

CLINICAL PRESENTATIONS

The most common presenting signs and symptoms of acute cystitis include dysuria, urgency, frequency, urinary urgency, bladder fullness, lower abdominal discomfort, suprapubic tenderness, and hematuria.[5] A patient may have one or more of these symptoms. The clinician should consider other diagnoses if a patient has systemic complaints.

DIAGNOSIS

The diagnosis of acute cystitis is made with a clean-catch urine specimen.[5] The urinalysis may show the presence of pyuria, microscopic hematuria, and/or positive nitrites. The urine culture must have more than 1000 CFU/mL. The pathogen or pathogens will be identified along with their corresponding antimicrobial sensitivities. Patients of reproductive age who are not known to be pregnant should always have a pregnancy test, as the choice of antibiotic for acute cystitis is dictated by the safety category for pregnancy.

TREATMENT

Treatment of acute cystitis involves empiric antibiotic therapy that covers the most common bacteria.[5] It is important for the clinician to be aware and consider local antimicrobial resistance patterns when prescribing antibiotics.

- Acute cystitis first-line agents for nonpregnant patients
  - Nitrofurantoin monohydrate
    - 100 mg by mouth 2 times a day × 5 days
  - Trimethoprim-sulfamethoxazole
    - 160 mg by mouth 2 times a day × 3 days
- Acute cystitis first-line agents for pregnancy
  - Cephalexin
    - 500 mg by mouth 2 times a day × 10 days
  - Nitrofurantoin monohydrate
    - 100 mg by mouth 2 times a day × 10 days
    - Avoid during the third trimester secondary to the risk of hemolytic disease of the newborn
  - Amoxicillin/clavulanate
    - 500 mg by mouth 2 times a day × 7 days
- Symptomatic care for acute cystitis
  - Phenazopyridine
    - 200 mg by mouth 2 times a day × 2 days

KEY POINTS

- Consider local antibiotic resistance patterns when prescribing empiric antibiotic therapy.[5]
- Obtain a pregnancy test before prescribing antibiotic therapy for acute cystitis, as some antibiotics can have teratogenic effects and are contraindicated in pregnancy.
- If prescribing phenazopyridine, educate the patient on adverse effects, specifically urine discoloration and contact lens staining.

ACUTE PYELONEPHRITIS

Acute pyelonephritis is defined as an upper UTI.[6] This means the causative organism responsible for the infection has ascended from the lower urinary tract to the kidney parenchyma. Clinical recognition of this disease state is important to avoid potentially life-threatening complications in both the nonpregnant and the pregnant patient, including sepsis, renal vein thrombosis, parenchymal renal scarring, renal failure, abscess formation, recurrent UTIs, or emphysematous pyelonephritis.

PATHOPHYSIOLOGY/CAUSE

The most common gram-negative bacterium associated with acute pyelonephritis is *E coli*.[6] Other responsible organisms in the pathogenesis of acute pyelonephritis include *Klebsiella*, *Enterobacter* species, *Proteus*, and gram-positive organisms. Bacteria ascend from the lower urinary tract and can exert effects on the kidney parenchyma, leading to poor perfusion to the kidneys, abscess formation, and scarring.

RISK FACTORS

Common risk factors associated with acute pyelonephritis include immunosuppression, recent urinary tract instrumentation, recent antibiotic use, and advanced age.[6]

CLINICAL PRESENTATIONS

Common presenting signs and symptoms of pyelonephritis include urinary urgency, urinary frequency, bladder fullness, lower abdominal discomfort, suprapubic tenderness, flank pain, costovertebral (CVA) tenderness, fevers, chills, malaise, nausea, vomiting, and hematuria.[6] The classic triad of fever, nausea and vomiting, and flank pain may or may not be present. Flank pain, CVA tenderness, fevers, chills, malaise, nausea, and vomiting are typically absent in acute cystitis.

DIAGNOSIS

Differential diagnoses associated with acute pyelonephritis include pelvic inflammatory disease (PID), acute cystitis, chronic pyelonephritis, nephrolithiasis, and pelvic pain syndrome.[6] The diagnosis of acute pyelonephritis requires a clean-catch urine specimen. The urinalysis may show the presence of pyuria, microscopic or gross hematuria, and/or positive nitrites. The urine culture must have more than 100,000 CFU, and the pathogen responsible for the underlying infection will be present. It is important to also obtain a urine pregnancy test, as the disposition of the patient and choice of antibiotic change with acute pyelonephritis in pregnancy. A complete blood count will likely demonstrate a leukocytosis, which can be infectious as well as inflammatory in nature. A complete metabolic panel should be ordered to determine if there are any electrolyte disturbances as well as to ensure renal functionality. If there is any renal insufficiency secondary to the diagnosis, further evaluation is warranted. Imaging may be indicated if a patient does not show clinical improvement despite appropriate antibiotic therapy. A computed tomography of the abdomen and pelvis may be ordered to help identify if there are any renal parenchymal perfusion changes, if there is any abscess formation, and to evaluate for perinephric fluid. A renal ultrasound can be ordered to evaluate for hydronephrosis secondary to an obstructive cause.

TREATMENT

Treatment of acute pyelonephritis involves empiric antibiotic therapy that covers gram-negative bacteria.[3,6–8] The most common bacterium is *E coli.* Other organisms that can cause acute pyelonephritis include *Proteus*, *Klebsiella*, and *Enterobacter* spp. It is important for the clinician to be aware and consider local antimicrobial resistance patterns when prescribing antibiotics. General guidelines are described here, but the clinician should identify that management of acute pyelonephritis is determined on an individual case-by-case assessment. In addition, patients who are immunocompromised, patients who have had an organ transplant, patients who have uncontrolled diabetes, and elderly patients usually require intravenous (IV) antibiotics. Other indications for hospitalization include inability to maintain oral hydration, hypotension, vomiting, dehydration, sepsis, comorbidities, the immunocompromised patient, and the pregnant patient.

- Several antibiotic regimens can be used for nonpregnant patients with acute uncomplicated pyelonephritis who can tolerate oral fluids and are considered hemodynamically stable and include the following:
  - Trimethoprim-sulfamethoxazole *or*
    - 160 mg by mouth 2 times a day × 14 days
  - Ciprofloxacin *or*
    - 500 mg by mouth 2 times a day × 5 to 7 days
  - Amoxicillin-clavulanate
    - 500 mg by mouth 2 times a day × 14 days
      - *Plus* ceftriaxone 1 g IV × 1
- First-line treatment of acute pyelonephritis in nonpregnant patients requiring inpatient therapy secondary to dehydration, inability to tolerate oral medications, and who are hemodynamically unstable includes IV hydration and antibiotics.
  - Ceftriaxone 1 g IV once daily *or*
  - Ciprofloxacin 400 mg IV every 12 hours *or*
  - Piperacillin/tazobactam 3.375 to 4.5 g IV every 6 hours *or* Meropenem 1 g IV every 8 hours *or* Ertapenem 1 g IV every 24 hours
- Hydration therapy in pyelonephritis
  - Once a patient is able to tolerate fluids by mouth and is hemodynamically stable, the patient can be converted to an appropriate oral regimen based on the urine culture and sensitivities. Until then, IV fluids are necessary to maintain adequate hydration of the renal parenchyma.
- If concern for enterococci infection is suspected, alternative antibiotic regimens must be selected for appropriate coverage against the gram-positive, anaerobic cocci, particularly in the hospital or other institutionalized setting.
  - Oral regimens include the following:
    - Amoxicillin 500 mg by mouth every 8 hours *or*
    - Amoxicillin/clavulanate (Augmentin) 875/125 mg by mouth 2 times a day *or*
    - Cefixime 400 mg by mouth daily *or*
    - Cefpodoxime 200 mg by mouth 2 times a day
  - IV regimens include the following:
    - Ampicillin 2 g IV every 4 hours *or*
    - Piperacillin/tazobactam 3.375 to 4.5 g every 6 hours *or*
    - Ceftriaxone 1 g IV every 24 hours *or*
    - Cefepime 1 to 2 g IV every 8 to 12 hours *or*
    - Ceftolozane-tazobactam 1.5 g IV every 8 hours *or*
    - Meropenem 1 g IV every 8 hours

- First-line treatment of acute pyelonephritis in pregnant patients requiring inpatient therapy includes IV hydration and antibiotics.
  - Mild to moderate pyelonephritis
    - Ceftriaxone (Rocephin) 1 g IV every 24 hours *or*
    - Cefepime (Maxipime) 1 g IV every 12 hours *or*
    - Cefotaxime (Claforan) 1 to 2 g IV every 8 hours *or*
    - Ceftazidime (Fortaz, Tazicef) 2 g IV every 8 hours *or*
    - Ampicillin 1 to 2 g IV every 6 hours *plus* gentamicin IV 1.5 mg/kg every 8 hours
  - Severe pyelonephritis
    - Ticarcillin-clavulanate (Timentin) 3.1 g IV every 6 hours *or*
    - Ampicillin-sulbactam (Unasyn) 1.5 g IV every 6 hours *or*
    - Piperacillin-tazobactam (Zosyn) 3.375 g IV every 6 hours
  - Once the patient is able to tolerate fluids by mouth and is hemodynamically stable, the patient can be converted to an appropriate oral regimen based on the urine culture and sensitivities.
- Antipyretic use
  - In pregnancy
    - Acetaminophen is the first-line treatment for antipyretic use throughout pregnancy.
    - Pregnant patients should avoid nonsteroidal anti-inflammatory drugs (NSAIDs) during pregnancy secondary to increase risk for miscarriage.
  - In the nonpregnant patient, acetaminophen and/or NSAIDs can be used.
- Hydration

KEY POINTS

- Consider local antibiotic resistance patterns when prescribing empiric antibiotic therapy.[6]
- The course of treatment for acute uncomplicated pyelonephritis is typically 2 weeks.

GROUP B STREPTOCOCCUS

Group B *Streptococcus* (GBS) is a gram-positive bacterium that is nonpathogenic in the nonpregnant patient. Clinical recognition of this disease during pregnancy is critical because of the significant harm if vertical transmission occurs during labor or after rupture of membranes, as GBS is the leading cause of newborn infection (ie, GBS meningitis, sepsis, UTI, pneumonia).[9]

PATHOPHYSIOLOGY/CAUSE

GBS is a gram-positive bacterium that can colonize in the gastrointestinal tract, perineum, and vagina.[9] Vertical transmission occurs during labor or after rupture of membranes.

EPIDEMIOLOGY

Common risk factors associated with GBS include gestational age less than 37 weeks, low birth weight, prolonged rupture of membranes, young maternal age, preterm prelabor rupture of membranes, and maternal black race.[9]

CLINICAL PRESENTATION

Patients who are found to be GBS positive through screening are asymptomatic.[9] Fever in the newborn within the first 90 days of life in a GBS-positive mother is concerning for vertical transmission of GBS to the newborn. GBS is not commonly tested for in the nonpregnant patient.

DIAGNOSIS

GBS is diagnosed through universal prenatal screening between 36 and 37 weeks via vaginal-rectal swab.[9] Patients may have had a urine culture earlier in pregnancy showing the presence of GBS.

TREATMENT IN PREGNANCY

Treatment of GBS includes intrapartum antibiotic prophylaxis for any patient that is GBS positive or if their GBS status is unknown at the time of labor, with the exception of a patient with a scheduled cesarean delivery with intact membranes.[9] This is because the GBS-positive neonate is at risk for GBS meningitis, sepsis, UTI, and pneumonia. Patients who have had GBS on urine culture should not be given oral antibiotics during pregnancy because it is likely recolonization will occur. Thus, they will be considered to be GBS positive when presenting to labor and delivery.

First-line antibiotic treatment of GBS is with penicillin G, 5 million units IV × 1 for the initial dose and then 2 to 4 million units IV every 4 hours until the infant is delivered. Treatment is most effective if Penicillin G is administered at least 4 hours before delivery. If the patient has a history of a penicillin allergy, but low risk of an immunoglobulin E–mediated response, then Cefazolin 2 g IV × 1 should be given for initial dose, and then 1 g IV every 8 hours until delivery. If the patient has a history of penicillin allergy, then they should receive Clindamycin 900 mg IV every 8 hours until delivery.

Patients should be educated and informed of their GBS status as soon as it is known and the requirements for prophylactic antibiotics. Patients should also be educated that GBS is not a sexually transmitted disease and is nonpathogenic to the pregnant patient.

KEY POINTS

- Intrapartum antibiotic treatment and prophylaxis are the mainstay of therapy.[9]
- Universal prenatal screening is key to effective prevention of GBS.
- Treatment during labor and delivery is aimed at preventing infection of the newborn.
- GBS is the leading cause of newborn infection (ie, GBS meningitis, sepsis, UTI, pneumonia).

VAGINITIS

Vaginitis is the most common gynecologic complaint seen in the office setting and thus an important diagnosis for the provider to know and be able to treat properly in both the nonpregnant and the pregnant patient to avoid unnecessary complications.[10,11] Defined as inflammation of the vagina, vaginitis has both infectious and noninfectious causes. Common infectious causes include bacterial vaginosis (BV), vaginal candidiasis, and trichomoniasis. The most common noninfectious causes encountered in the clinical setting including allergic reaction, irritation, and atrophic vaginitis secondary to estrogen deficiency.

The clinical presentation of vaginitis can differ based on the underlying cause. The clinician should assess for a large spectrum of vaginal symptoms, including abnormal discharge, vulvovaginal discomfort, vaginal malodor, vaginal and vulvar itching, dyspareunia, and dysuria.

The clinician should perform a complete pelvic examination in all patients suspected of having vaginitis. The vulva, vagina, and cervix should be assessed for friability, erythema, lesions, and discharge. Vaginal mucosa that is pale and shiny with loss of rugae is likely atrophic vaginitis. Specific laboratory studies may include saline and potassium hydroxide wet mount, whiff test, pH testing, vaginal culture, and/or nucleic acid amplification testing. Specific findings are discussed later.

BACTERIAL VAGINOSIS

Bacterial vaginosis (BV) has a high prevalence in both the nonpregnant and the pregnant patient population and is the most common cause of vaginitis in the symptomatic patient.[10–12] In addition, pregnant patients with BV have a higher risk of preterm labor and spontaneous abortion, making the diagnosis and treatment of BV important in the pregnant patient.

PATHOPHYSIOLOGY/CAUSE

BV is a common cause of vaginal discharge in the pregnant patient secondary to the vaginal pH changes that occur owing to hormonal influences.[10,11] BV results from a microbial alteration or disturbance away from the common *Lactobacillus* species to anaerobic bacteria, which ultimately alters the vaginal flora and leads to overgrowth of pathogens. *Gardnerella vaginalis* is the most common pathogen involved. The altered microbial milieu results in an increase in vaginal pH > 4.5, and symptoms may become apparent.

RISK FACTORS

Common risk factors associated with BV include multiple sex partners, douching, cigarette smoking, PID, copper-containing intrauterine devices, damp or tight-fitting clothing, scented detergents and soaps, poor hygiene, and the presence of other sexually transmitted infections (STIs), specifically herpes simplex virus (HSV) type 2, gonorrhea, chlamydia, trichomonas, and HIV.[10,11] Lesbian patients are also at greater risk of developing BV.

CLINICAL PRESENTATION

The clinical presentation of BV can be asymptomatic or symptomatic.[10,11] If patients are symptomatic, they will experience milky thin grayish white vaginal discharge that may or may not be odorous. The specific odor of BV, if present, is classically described as "fishy," resulting from amine production.

DIAGNOSIS

The diagnosis of BV can be clinical and confirmed through laboratory testing.[10,11] The Amsel criteria (**Table 1**) can be used to diagnose BV. It requires the patient to have 3 out of 4 criteria to be present to confidently diagnosis BV.

Table 1	
The Amsel criteria	
Vaginal discharge	Homogenous, milky, white, thin in appearance
pH (of vaginal fluid)	>4.5 (normal 3.8–4.2)
Saline wet mount	Presence of clue cells on microscopic examination
Positive whiff test	Fishy odor (amine odor) of vaginal discharge after addition of 10% potassium hydroxide

The saline wet mount for BV will have the presence of "clue cells." Clue cells are vaginal epithelial cells covered with rods and cocci bacteria, creating a stippled or granular appearance. A decreased number of lactobacilli are observed, and white blood cells are absent unless a secondary infection is present.

TREATMENT

Indication for treatment of BV is to relieve symptoms, reduce signs of infection, and decrease the risk of acquiring HIV and/or other STIs.[10–12]

- Nonpregnant first-line therapy for BV is metronidazole 500 mg by mouth 2 times a day × 7 days. Second-line treatment is tinidazole 2 g by mouth daily × 2 days or 1 g by mouth daily × 5 days. Metronidazole 500 mg by mouth 2 times a day × 7 days is the treatment of choice in the second and third trimesters of pregnancy. Metronidazole and tinidazole should be avoiding in the first trimester because it crosses the placenta, creating a potential risk for teratogenicity. An alternative regimen is clindamycin 300 mg by mouth 2 times a day × 7 days. Patient education includes refraining from sexual activity during treatment and avoiding douching.
- Recurrent BV is fairly common. This is likely due to failure of the antibiotic to eradicate the overgrowth of the pathogens and disruption of the vaginal flora away from the common *Lactobacillus* species, inconsistent condom use, and resuming sexual intercourse with partner following antibiotic treatment. Treatment of recurrent BV with a long-term suppressive regimen includes metronidazole vaginal 0.75% gel intravaginal twice a week for 4 to 6 months after treatment with metronidazole, tinidazole, or clindamycin. Adding intravaginal boric acid suppositories to the suppression regimen may be beneficial.
- Postcoital BV transmission is highly prevalent, and treatment of the partner is favored in particular for women who have sex with women. It is thought that consistent use of condoms and male circumcision help reduce the risk of BV in women who have sex with men. Treatment regimens for postcoital BV include metronidazole 500 mg by mouth 2 times a day × 7 days, tinidazole 2 g by mouth daily × 2 days, or 1 g by mouth daily × 5 days, or clindamycin 300 mg by mouth 2 times a day × 7 days.

KEY POINTS

- Pregnant patients with BV have a higher risk of preterm labor.[10,11]
- Metronidazole 500 mg by mouth 2 times a day × 7 days is the treatment of choice in the second and third trimesters of pregnancy.
- Metronidazole and tinidazole should be avoiding in the first trimester because it crosses the placenta, creating a potential risk for teratogenicity.

- Avoid alcohol consumption when taking metronidazole secondary to a disulfiram-like reaction that can occur, which presents as abdominal pain, nausea, vomiting, headache, and seizures.
- Avoid breastfeeding while taking metronidazole.

VAGINAL CANDIDIASIS

Vaginal candidiasis has a high prevalence in both the nonpregnant and the pregnant patient population and is the second most common cause of vaginitis in the symptomatic patient.[11]

PATHOPHYSIOLOGY/CAUSE

Vaginal candidiasis occurs when there is a disturbance of the vaginal pH, which ultimately alters the vaginal flora and leads to overgrowth of pathogens.[11] The most common cause of vaginal candidiasis is the *Candida* species. *Candida albicans* accounts for 85% to 90% cases of vaginal candidiasis.

RISK FACTORS

Common risk factors associated with vaginal candidiasis are pregnancy, combined hormonal contraceptive use, chronic corticosteroid use, intrauterine device use, intercourse at a young age, increased frequency of intercourse, diabetes, immunocompromised states, long-term antibiotic use, recent antibiotic use, damp or tight-fitting clothing, and poor hygiene.[11]

CLINICAL MANIFESTATIONS

The clinical manifestations of vaginal candidiasis are pruritus; a thick, white, curdlike vaginal discharge; vulva erythema with or without satellite lesions; vulvar dyspareunia; vulvar burning; and a normal-appearing cervix. Pruritus is frequently the most common complaint in patients with vaginal candidiasis.[11]

DIAGNOSIS

Vaginal candidiasis can be diagnosed clinically and confirmed with a saline wet mount, which will show hyphae and budding yeast. In addition, in general, Candida infections will present with a normal pH of less than 4.5 (**Table 2**).[11]

TREATMENT

Treatment of vaginal candidiasis is with an oral or vaginal antifungal.[11,13] First-line oral therapy is fluconazole 150 mg by mouth 1 time. Sometimes patients will need to repeat the dose in a few days if symptoms persist. Fluconazole is contraindicated in pregnancy and is only available by prescription. Intravaginal antifungals include clotrimazole 1% cream, miconazole 2% cream, and tioconazole 6.5%. Intravaginal preparations are available over the counter. In addition, the use of intravaginal boric

Table 2		
pH for vaginitis causes		
Bacterial Vaginosis	Vaginal Candidiasis	Trichomonas
5.0–6.0	<4.5	5.0–7.0

acid for 10 to 14 days for women who are azole resistant has been shown to be effective in recurrent vaginal candidiasis.

KEY POINTS

- Pruritus is the most common presenting complaint.[11]
- Oral fluconazole is contraindicated in pregnancy.

TRICHOMONIASIS

Trichomoniasis is the third most common cause of vaginitis.[11,14] Trichomoniasis is a sexually transmitted disease. Infection of trichomoniasis during pregnancy can cause preterm delivery and/or low-birth-weight infants.

PATHOPHYSIOLOGY/CAUSE

Trichomoniasis is caused when there is a disturbance of the vaginal pH, which ultimately alters the vaginal flora and leads to overgrowth of pathogens.[11,14] Trichomoniasis is caused by the flagellated protozoa *Trichomonas vaginalis*.

RISK FACTORS

Common risk factors associated with trichomoniasis include tobacco use, unprotected intercourse, multiple sex partners, intrauterine device use, and the presence of other STIs.[11,14]

CLINICAL MANIFESTATIONS

Clinical manifestations associated with trichomoniasis include punctate lesions on the cervix, which is coined a "strawberry cervix."[11,14] In addition, these patients can have a copious, frothy, discharge that can be gray, yellow, white, or green in color. Patients may complain of postcoital bleeding as well.

DIAGNOSIS

The diagnosis of vaginal trichomoniasis requires the presence of motile protozoans on a saline wet mount or through polymerase chain reaction (PCR) testing.[11,14] In addition, in general, trichomonas will present with an elevated pH of between 5.0 and 7.0 (see **Table 2**).

TREATMENT

Treatment of trichomoniasis requires the use of oral antiprotozoals.[11,14] Metronidazole 2 g by mouth 1 time is the preferred regimen. Metronidazole is considered first line in both the pregnant and the nonpregnant woman, with the exception of the lactating woman and a woman in her first trimester. Tinidazole 2 g by mouth as a single dose is an effective alternative treatment regimen. Sexual partners of patients with a diagnosis of trichomoniasis should be treated and offered STI screening. In addition, patients should avoid sexual contact until they and their sexual partner or partners are cured.

KEY POINTS

- Infection during pregnancy can cause preterm delivery and/or low-birth-weight infants.[11,14]

- Avoid alcohol consumption when taking metronidazole secondary to a disulfiram-like reaction that can occur, which presents as abdominal pain, nausea, vomiting, headache, and seizures.
- Avoid breastfeeding while taking metronidazole.

CERVICITIS

Cervicitis has multiple causes, including noninfectious and infectious causes.[15] STIs are the most common causes of cervicitis, with chlamydia being the most prevalent, followed by gonorrhea. Untreated cervicitis can lead to PID, and untreated cervicitis in the pregnant patient can cause preterm labor and is a risk factor for early pregnancy loss.

PATHOPHYSIOLOGY/CAUSE

The most common causes of cervicitis are *Chlamydia trachomatis* and *Neisseria gonorrhoeae*.[15] Another common cause is HSV.

RISK FACTORS

Common risk factors associated with cervicitis include multiple sex partners, young age, a history of sexually transmitted disease, and pregnancy.[15]

CLINICAL PRESENTATIONS

Clinical manifestations associated with cervicitis include abnormal vaginal discharge, intermenstrual vaginal bleeding, postcoital bleeding, and dysuria.[15,16] Some individuals may be asymptomatic until a pelvic examination is performed, causing pain with the speculum examination or on bimanual examination.

DIAGNOSIS

A presumptive diagnosis of cervicitis can be made if the cervix appears erythematous, edematous, and easily friable.[16] Definitive diagnosis is through microbial testing with PCR or nucleic acid amplification testing. If the patient is experiencing fever and cervical motion tenderness, a presumptive diagnosis of PID should be made and empiric therapy initiated.

TREATMENT

First-line treatment of *C trachomatis* is doxycycline 100 mg orally twice a day for 7 days.[15–17] Azithromycin can be used as an alternative for those unable to take doxycycline.

First-line treatment of gonorrhea is ceftriaxone 250 mg intramuscular injection in a single dose. Whenever chlamydia or gonorrhea is suspected, both doxycycline and ceftriaxone should be used.

First-line treatment of HSV is acyclovir 400 mg by mouth 3 times daily × 7 to 10 days, valacyclovir 1000 mg by mouth twice daily × 7 to 10 days, or famciclovir 250 mg by mouth 3 times daily × 7 to 10 days.

Patients should be educated to abstain from sexual intercourse until they have completed the full course of treatment and their partner is tested and treated. Inadequately treated chlamydial or gonorrheal infections can lead to PID. The data do not support routine tests of cure unless the patient is pregnant; however, if compliance is questioned or known reinfection occurs, test of cure (TOC) is appropriate.[3] The current recommendation for a TOC is no less than 4 weeks after treatment.[3]

All patients with STIs should be offered additional testing for HIV and syphilis, specifically if risk factors exist.

KEY POINTS

- If left untreated, cervicitis can lead to PID.
- It is important to treat for cervicitis in the pregnant patient to avoid the risk of preterm labor and/or miscarriage.

REFERENCES

1. Lerma Edgar. Asymptomatic bacteriuria. Available at: https://emedicine. medscape.com/article/2059290-overview. Accessed July 15, 2021.
2. US Preventive Services Task Force. Screening for asymptomatic bacteriuria in adults: US Preventive Services Task Force recommendation statement. JAMA 2019;322(12):1188–94.
3. Fulop, Tibor. Acute pyelonephritis treatment & management. Updated July 1, 2021. Accessed September 5, 2021.
4. Jin J. Screening for asymptomatic bacteriuria. JAMA 2019;322(12):1222.
5. Brusch John. Urinary tract infection (UTI) and cystitis (bladder infection) in females. Available at: https://emedicine.medscape.com/article/233101-overview. Accessed July 20, 2021.
6. Fulop, Tibor. Acute pyelonephritis. Available at: https://emedicine.medscape. com/article/245559-overview. Accessed July 15, 2021.
7. Yau, Amy. Available at: https://emedicine.medscape.com/article/2002753-overview. Accessed September 6, 2021.
8. Bremer L, Golctzke J, Wiessner C, et al. Paracetamol medication during pregnancy: insights on intake frequencies, dosages and effects on hematopoietic stem cell populations in cord blood from a longitudinal prospective pregnancy cohort. EBioMedicine 2017;26:146–51.
9. American College of Obstetricians and Gynecologists. ACOG Practice Bulletin no. 797. Prevention of Group B Streptococcal Early-Onset Disease in Newborns. June 2019
10. Center for Disease Control and Prevention. 2021 sexually transmitted infections treatment guidelines. 2021. Available at: https://www.cdc.gov/std/treatment-guidelines/bv.htm.
11. Gor HB. Vaginitis. Available at: https://emedicine.medscape.com/article/257141-overview. Accessed July 20, 2021.
12. Barbieri R. Effective treatment of recurrent bacterial vaginosis. 2017 [online] Mdedge.com. Available at: https://www.mdedge.com/obgyn/article/141388/gynecology/effective-treatment-recurrent-bacterial-vaginosis. Accessed 8 September 2021.
13. Powell A, Ghanem KG, Rogers L, et al. Clinicians' use of intravaginal boric acid maintenance therapy for recurrent vulvovaginal candidiasis and bacterial vaginosis. Sex Transm Dis 2019;46(12):810–2.
14. Workowski KA, Bachmann LH, Chang PA, et al. Sexually transmitted infections treatment guidelines, 2021. MMWR Recomm Rep 2021;70(No. 4):1–187.

15. Centers for Disease Control and Prevention. 2021 disease characterized by urethritis and cervicitis. 2021. Available at: https://www.cdc.gov/std/treatment-guidelines/urethritis-and-cervicitis.htm. Accessed September 8, 2021.

16. Ollendorff AT. Cervicitis. Available at: https://emedicine.medscape.com/article/253402-overview. Accessed September 8, 2021.

17. Centers for Disease Control and Prevention. Sexually transmitted infections guidelines, 2021. Chlamydia. Available at: https://www.cdc.gov/std/treatment-guidelines/chlamydia.htm. Accessed September 8, 2021.

Breast Cancer

Ami Robinson Steele, DMSc, PA-C, DFAAPA[a],*,
Elyse Watkins, DHSc, PA-C, DFAAPA, NCMP[b,c]

KEYWORDS

- Breast • Cancer • Adenocarcinoma • Carcinoma in situ • Invasive carcinoma
- Mastectomy • Breast-conserving • Aromatase inhibitor • Tamoxifen • survivorship

KEY POINTS

- The most common breast malignancies are estrogen and progesterone receptor positive and human epidermal growth factor receptor (HER2) negative, thus having a better overall survival.
- Risk factors for breast cancer vary from family history, genetics, and hormonal influences to lifestyle impacts.
- Treatment options include chemotherapeutic treatment based on the molecular profile and stage of breast cancer. Surgical interventions such as breast-conserving surgery or mastectomy depend on the stage and risk for recurrence. Patient expectations and desires are also considered.
- Screening for breast cancer is imperative for early diagnosis and intervention.
- Survivorship considers the journey of the patient with breast cancer from diagnosis, through treatment, and throughout the rest of their life.

INTRODUCTION

Breast cancer is the second leading cause of cancer deaths in women.[1] It is estimated that 1 in 8 women will be diagnosed in their lifetime, or up to 284,000 annually.[1,2] Nearly 50,000 women will be diagnosed with stage 0 breast cancer, also known as carcinoma in situ. Still, more than 40,000 will succumb to the disease each year.[1] Patient education, a clear understanding of disease presentation related to the breast cancer subtype, risk factors, diagnosis, treatment strategies, and survivorship is imperative for health-care providers to impart to patients. As there are nearly 4 million breast cancer survivors in the United States, we must strengthen our partnership with patients in both screening, diagnosis, and surveillance. However, this article will not specifically focus on early-onset breast cancer.

[a] Department of Physician Assistant Studies, College of Health Sciences, Gardner-Webb University, PO Box 7252, Boiling Springs, NC 28017, USA; [b] University of Lynchburg School of PA Medicine, 1501 Lakeside Drive, Lynchburg, VA 24501, USA; [c] Florida State University School of PA Practice, 1115 W Call Street, Tallahassee, FL 32304, USA
* Corresponding author.
E-mail address: ami.steele@yahoo.com

Physician Assist Clin 7 (2022) 433–445
https://doi.org/10.1016/j.cpha.2022.03.002
2405-7991/22/© 2022 Elsevier Inc. All rights reserved.

DISCUSSION
Risk Factors

Although each subset of breast cancer is unique, the general risk factors for developing breast cancer are related to gender, age, lifestyle, genetics, and family history. Women are diagnosed with breast cancer far more often than men. As women age, the risk of developing breast cancer increases. According to the American Cancer Society (ACS), 1:8 invasive breast cancers develop in women aged younger than 45 years, whereas 2:3 invasive breast cancers are found in women aged 55 years or older.[3]

Known genetic history, family history, or personal history of cancer are all risk factors. According to the ACS, 5% to 10% of breast cancers are likely hereditary in which gene mutations are inherited, including the more common breast cancer gene (BRCA) 1 and BRCA2 mutations.[3] Additional genetic mutations exist but are less common.[3] Having a first-degree relative with breast cancer doubles the risk, whereas a 3-fold increase in risk exists in women with 2 or more first-degree relatives who have had breast cancer.[3] Up to 25% of women with breast cancer have a family member who has been diagnosed with breast cancer as well.[3,4] Patients who present with carcinoma in situ or invasive carcinoma should be referred for genetic counseling and testing.

Further risk factors are directly related to the lifetime physiologic impact of estrogen. The onset of menses before the age of 12 years, nulliparity, or first pregnancy after 30 years of age contribute to an increased risk of breast cancer because plasma estrogen is circulating much longer in these women. Because breastfeeding diminishes the number of overall menstrual cycles in a woman's lifetime, those who do not breastfeed are slightly more at risk. The use of combined hormonal contraception is also associated with a slightly increased risk of breast cancer development that returns to normal within 10 years of discontinuation.[3] Hormone replacement therapy (HRT) is often used in menopausal patients to relieve the symptoms associated with menopause. After 4 years of use, combined hormone therapy confers an increased risk in the presence of cancer and the likelihood it will be diagnosed at an advanced stage.[3] Within 5 years of discontinuing combined hormone therapy, the risk of breast cancer returns to normal.[3] Breast cancer survivors who take HRT are at greater risk of cancer recurrence.[4] Patients who enter menopause after 55 years of age have an increased risk of developing breast cancer.

Lifestyle strongly influences breast cancer development. Weight and physical activity contribute to risks of breast cancer development. Obesity body mass index (BMI >25) and a sedentary lifestyle are known risk factors. Postmenopausal obesity is associated with an increased risk of hormone-receptor-positive breast cancer, whereas premenopausal obesity is associated with a higher risk of triple-negative breast cancer development.[3] A sedentary lifestyle carries an increased risk of developing breast cancer compared with an active one. Increased physical activity will diminish both the risk of developing breast cancer as well as its recurrence. Drinking alcohol-containing beverages can stimulate estrogen receptors.[4] Therefore, women who consume 2 to 3 alcoholic beverages daily have a 20% greater chance of developing breast cancer than those who do not drink alcohol.[3] Early-aged smoking confers a higher risk of breast cancer development.[4] Excessive dietary fat intake, particularly saturated fat, leads to a poor prognosis and a higher mortality rate in patients diagnosed with breast cancer.[4]

Additional risk factors include dense breast tissue, which increases the risk of breast cancer by 1.5 to 2-fold. In addition, exposure to diethylstilbestrol or previous chest radiation as a teen or young adult contributes to increased risk. Finally, although White women are slightly more likely to develop breast cancer overall, Black women aged younger than 45 years are more likely to develop breast cancer than White women in the same age group and have worse outcomes.[3,4]

Clinical Presentation

Although it is no longer recommended that patients conduct monthly self-breast examinations, an understanding of normal breast tissue for the individual remains essential to discuss with each patient. As expected, the most common presentation of breast cancer is a patient finding a mass or lump in the breast. Although these are often associated with benign breast disorders, the pursuit of a definitive diagnosis is imperative for each patient. Masses associated with breast carcinoma are more often immobile, painless, and have poorly defined margins. Cancerous breast masses are primarily painless, but the adage that cancer is painless does not apply to all breast cancers. Some patients will complain of breast tenderness associated with the mass, making it essential to never eliminate the possibility of cancer based on the presence of pain.

Additional common presenting symptoms include edema of the breast, nipple changes (everted to inverted), nipple discharge, nipple pain, retractions in the breast parenchyma, and skin dimpling. In advanced disease, axillary lymphadenopathy may be palpable. However, invasive breast cancer and carcinoma in situ are often diagnosed on routine screening mammography in asymptomatic patients.

Breast Cancer Types and Molecular Subtypes

Identifying the type and subtype of the area of concern is fundamental to diagnostic and therapeutic approaches. Generally, breast cancers are either adenocarcinomas or other less common types that arise from different cells. Adenocarcinomas of the breast arise from the glandular cells lining the ducts or lobules.[5,6] Adenocarcinomas are either in situ or invasive. Other types of breast cancers, not adenocarcinomas, are far less common, invasive, and require specific types of treatment.[6] This article will focus on the more common types.

In situ adenocarcinoma

Ductal carcinoma in situ. Ductal carcinoma in situ (DCIS) is also known as stage 0 breast adenocarcinoma. It is a precancerous overgrowth of atypical cells lining the mammary ducts without invading beyond the ductal walls into the nearby breast tissue.[7] It is a clinically silent disease because of the absence of physical examination findings associated with DCIS. Although noninvasive, it can grow and metastasize over time as a nonobligate precursor of invasive breast cancer.[8] Studies have found that at least 30% of DCIS cases will advance to invasive disease over several decades.[8] Less commonly, it can be associated with overlying Paget disease.[9] DCIS accounts for 1 in 5 new breast malignant diagnoses but has a very high cure rate. Risk factors align with those previously mentioned. Intervention for DCIS is either breast-conserving surgery (BCS) +/− radiation or simple mastectomy.[7,9] BCS is also known as lumpectomy. Mastectomy may be more appropriate for more extensive lesions, but ultimately the patient and the surgeon decide on the most appropriate surgical intervention. Hormonally responsive lesions, also known as hormone receptor positive, are treated with hormone-blocking therapy after surgery.[7,9] Either way, sentinel lymph node biopsy may accompany BCS or mastectomy.[7]

Lobular carcinoma in situ. Lobular carcinoma in situ (LCIS) is a precancerous growth of atypical lobular cells.[9] Although DCIS is far more common, the incidence of LCIS is increasing. LCIS is associated with an increased risk of breast cancer developing in the ipsilateral or contralateral breast. Antiestrogen hormone therapy is the most effective prevention of the development of invasive breast cancer, but some patients may opt for prophylactic lumpectomy or mastectomy.[9]

Invasive adenocarcinoma

Invasive lobular carcinoma. Invasive lobular carcinoma (ILC) accounts for up to 10% of all invasive breast cancers.[10] Although it is less common than invasive ductal carcinoma (IDC), it is more likely to occur in postmenopausal women due to their advanced age.[10] It is most often hormonally mediated, producing estrogen/progesterone-positive, HER2-negative tumors. ILC tumors are often large with ill-defined margins but not detectable as palpable lesions on clinical presentation. Bilateral ILC is also more common than in IDC, with an occurrence rate of 10% to 20%. Distant metastases are more often found in gastrointestinal or peritoneal sites.[10]

Invasive ductal carcinoma. The most common breast cancer is IDC, accounting for 70% to 80% of invasive breast carcinoma diagnoses.[11] Similar to the precancerous DCIS, IDC originates in the mammary ducts, invading the duct walls and nearby structures, thus making it invasive.

Other breast cancers

Paget disease of the breast. One percent of breast cancer is Paget disease of the breast. The skin changes associated with Paget disease include eczematous changes that alter the nipple, areola, and surrounding skin that may also be thickened, crusted, and have pigmentation changes. Patients often complain of associated discomfort (pain or burning) and pruritis. Diagnosis is usually made based on the histologic finding of Paget cells on biopsy. About 85% of patients with Paget disease will have a DCIS or IDC as well.[9]

Inflammatory breast cancer. Inflammatory breast cancer is characterized by sudden skin changes, including indurated, dimpled skin (peau d'orange), erythema, and pain.[9] Inflammatory breast cancer has a poor prognosis and should be a consideration in a patient with mastitis that does not resolve with appropriate antimicrobial therapy.

Angiosarcoma. Angiosarcoma (AS) arises from the endothelial cells of blood and lymphatic vessels, often as a subsequent complication of previous breast radiotherapy within the last 8 to 10 years.[12] Less than 1% of breast malignancies will be AS. AS present as skin lesions that seem to be plaques or patches.[13] Primary AS arises in nonirradiated women, typically in their 30s to 40s. Secondary AS seems in older women who have had previous breast cancer radiation treatment. Although it occurs in the endothelial cells of blood and lymphatic cells, it may invade the breast tissue.[12,13] The 5-year survival rate for radiation-induced AS ranges from 28% to 54%. Mastectomy with negative margins is the standard treatment approach. Typically, lymph nodes are not dissected due to lack of involvement.[13] Due to the significant recurrence rate (54% to 92%), cotreatment with chemotherapy and radiation are more effective.[13] Most recurrences occur in the first postoperative year and are found most commonly along the mastectomy scar. Subsequent recurrences can be as high as 48%.[13]

Molecular Subtypes of Breast Cancer

There are 4 main molecular subtypes of breast cancer based on the tumor's genetic and immunohistochemical biomarkers. Tumors are classified according to their hormone (estrogen and progesterone) receptivity and overexpression of human epidermal growth factor receptor-2.

- *Luminal A*: Hormone receptor positive; HER-2 negative
- *Luminal B*: Hormone receptor positive; HER-2 positive
- *Triple negative (TNBC)*: Hormone receptor negative, HER-2 negative
  - ○ TNBC subclassification
    - Luminal androgen receptor
    - Mesenchymal-like
    - Immunomodulatory
    - Basal-like
- *HER2*: HER-2 positive, hormone receptor negative

TNBC breast cancers carry the worst prognosis, whereas Luminal A has the best prognosis. The reasons for these differences are varied, but generally, it is due to the lack of specific targets of treatment in TNBC. In addition, TNBC usually affects younger patients and is more aggressive than the other molecular subtypes.

Tissue that is biopsied will undergo immunohistologic biomarker analysis to help stratify risk and determine the next steps in management. Ultrasound-guided core needle biopsy of the suspicious area(s) is the preferred method of biopsy. Several genomic tests have been developed to help stratify a patient's risk of recurrence. The Oncotype DX is the most common, but not all oncologists use this to stratify risk because the evidence is mixed. However, see **Tables 1** and **2** for an outline of scoring.

Diagnostic Imaging

Mammography yields a sensitivity of 57% to 81%.[14] Ultrasound sensitivity is more remarkable than mammography, at 68% to 98%, leading to better accuracy in estimating tumor size but not necessarily initial diagnosis.[14] Breast magnetic resonance imaging carries a sensitivity of 93% to 96%.[14]

Medical Management

Management of breast cancer must consider multiple variables, including the molecular subtype, staging, the overall health of the patient, menopausal status, and the likelihood of achieving a disease-free status with the least likely chance of recurrence.

Table 1 Oncotype DX: Genomic Testing ≤50 y [14]	
Genomic Test to Inform Breast Cancer Treatment of Women aged less than 50 years.	
Oncotype DX Recurrence Score	**Treatment Approach**
0–15	1. Cancer has a low risk of recurrence. 2. The benefit of chemo does not outweigh the risks of side effects.
16–20	1. Cancer has a low-to-medium risk of recurrence. 2. The benefit of chemo will unlikely outweigh the risk of side effects.
21–25	1. Cancer has a medium risk of recurrence 2. The benefit of chemo will likely outweigh the side effects.
26–100	1. Cancer has a high risk of recurrence. 2. The benefit of chemo exceeds the risk of side effects.

Table 2
Oncotype DX: Genomic Testing >50 y [14]

Genomic Test to Inform Breast Cancer Treatment for Females > 50 years	
Oncotype DX Recurrence Score	Treatment Approach
0–25	1. Cancer has a low risk of recurrence. 2. The benefit of chemo does not outweigh the risks of side effects.
26–100	1. Cancer has a high risk of recurrence. 2. The benefit of chemo exceeds the risk of side effects.

Other considerations include the patient's desire for a future pregnancy and breast reconstruction. The balance of benefit and risk is key to the management approach for each patient.

Selective estrogen receptor modulators

Selective estrogen receptor modulators (SERMs) act as agonists or antagonists of estrogen receptors.[4] There are 2 types of SERMS. Tamoxifen is the most widely studied and most commonly prescribed SERM used to treat estrogen-receptor-positive breast cancers of all stages. It can be used as adjuvant or neoadjuvant therapy in treating breast cancer or as part of cancer prevention because of its success in reducing noninvasive and invasive breast cancer risks.[4] Although tamoxifen has demonstrated a significant reduction in estrogen-receptor (ER)-positive breast cancer after 5 years of treatment, there are substantial risks associated with its use.[4] Endometrial hyperplasia and cancer and thromboembolic events (stroke, pulmonary embolism, and deep-vein thrombosis) are potential side effects that warrant consideration of its benefits over potential risks.[4] Other possible complications for patients include fatty liver disease, ophthalmic disorders, hair thinning, vaginal dryness, discharge, bleeding, weight gain/edema, and hot flashes.[15–17] See **Table 3**. Despite the side effects and adverse events associated with its use, it is still considered first-line for premenopausal patients with hormone receptor positive breast cancer. SERMs are used as adjuvant therapy after the patient has had surgery and radiation. It is also indicated for prevention in patients at high risk of developing breast cancer.

Aromatase inhibitors

Aromatase inhibitors (AIs) treat estrogen-receptor-positive breast cancer in postmenopausal women by reducing plasma estrogen levels by disrupting estrogen biosynthesis from androgens.[4] Although used mainly in postmenopausal women, AIs can be prescribed for premenopausal women when coupled with ovarian suppression. There are 2 classes: a steroidal inhibitor (exemestane) and nonsteroidal inhibitors (anastrozole, letrozole).[4] Several studies have demonstrated more significant efficacy as adjuvant therapy in reducing breast cancer incidents as monotherapy and following 2 to 3 years of tamoxifen. Although tamoxifen has a more substantial side-effect profile, drawbacks exist with AIs.[4] **Table 3** provides a more detailed outline of the side effects of each therapy. The most significant side effect includes a greater risk of osteoporosis, leading to an increased risk of fractures.[4,16–19] AI-associated musculoskeletal syndrome (AIMSS) consists of the constellation of symptoms: arthralgia, joint stiffness, +/− bone pain, and carpal tunnel syndrome. In approximately 30% of patients,[16–18] AIMSS symptoms are severe enough to lead to AI discontinuation. Other

Table 3
Associated complications with breast cancer medical interventions

Health Issue	SERMs	AIs	MAs	Anthracyclines
Bone demineralization/osteoporosis	●	●		
Breathing difficulty/dyspnea	●			●
Cardiotoxicity (CHF, cardiomyopathy)	●		●	●
Depression	●	●		
Diarrhea			●	●
Fatigue	●	●		
Forgetfulness	●	●		
Alopecia	●			●
Liver disorder/damage	●		●	
MSK and joint pain	●	●		
Mood changes	●	●		
Nausea/vomiting	●			●
Sexual dysfunction/libido loss	●	●		
Sleep disturbances	●	●		
Vaginal dryness	●	●		
Vasomotor symptoms	●	●		

CHF, congestive heart failure; MSK, musculoskeletal.

complications include cardiovascular disease, diabetes, hypercholesterolemia, vaginal dryness, sexual dysfunction, insomnia, and forgetfulness.[16–18] AIs are used as adjuvant therapy after the patient has had surgery and radiation.

Monoclonal antibodies
Monoclonal antibodies (MAs) are artificial antibodies that attach to a specific target (eg, HER2 protein) and terminate cell growth.[20,21] Examples include trastuzumab, trastuzumab plus hyaluronidase injection, pertuzumab, and hyaluronidase, and margetuximab.[20] Other MAs are in development. Drug class side effects include cardiotoxicity, severe diarrhea, hand-foot syndrome, liver damage, and infusion-induced syndrome/cytokine storm. Cardiotoxicity occurs in 4% of women treated with trastuzumab.[20,21] It is described as an asymptomatic decrease in the left ventricular ejection fraction. There are 2 types: Type 1 is caused by cardiomyocyte necrosis or apoptosis and is irreversible and Type 2 is the result of cardiomyocyte dysfunction and is reversible with medication discontinuation.[20,21]

Chemotherapeutic medications
Anthracyclines (doxorubicin), taxanes (paclitaxel), platinum agents (cisplatin or carboplatin), and others are commonly used chemotherapeutic interventions as an adjuvant or neoadjuvant drug, particularly in TNBC. Administered intravenously as an infusion or injection, the side effects comprise a long list, including nausea/vomiting/diarrhea, alopecia, nail changes, mouth sores, anorexia, neuropathy, fatigue, hand-foot syndrome, and decrease in mental function. In addition, cardiotoxicity can occur. Cardiotoxicity encompasses left ventricular ejection fraction reduction and heart failure.[22–24] Myelosuppression that ranges from severe infection to septic shock to death can occur.[22–24] Myelodysplastic syndromes or acute myeloid leukemia can occur but are quite rare and generally manifest within 10 years of therapy.

Neoadjuvant systemic therapy

Neoadjuvant is therapy given before surgical intervention. With the primary goal of mass size-reduction facilitating more successful surgical intervention with BCS, or in the face of HER2-positive cancers, neoadjuvant systemic therapy may be initiated in patients. Examples of neoadjuvant treatments include chemotherapy, HER2-targeted drugs (eg, trastuzumab), or hormone therapies (SERMs and AIs). The treatment decision must consider the patient's age, the status of lymph node involvement, size of the tumor, comorbid conditions, and other immunohistologic testing, if applicable.[2]

The extent of disease spread largely determines the neoadjuvant and adjuvant therapy approaches.[25] If metastatic Stage IV breast cancer is confirmed, systemic therapy is the preferred approach unless resection of the primary tumor is necessary for pain reduction.[25]

Other indications for neoadjuvant chemotherapies include inflammatory breast cancer; bony chest wall tumor fixation; extensive skin involvement (ulceration or satellite skin nodules); and involvement of the axilla, including matted axillary lymphadenopathy, axillary neurovascular involvement, or lymphedema of the contralateral or ipsilateral upper extremity.[25] For a more complete outline of side effects and adverse events of chemotherapeutic options, see **Table 3**.

Radiation Therapy

Radiation therapy can be administered before surgery and is usually dependent on the size of the mass. For example, if a mass is large and debulking with radiation may help the surgeon remove the mass, neoadjuvant radiation will be considered. Most often, radiation therapy is administered postoperatively, once the wound has had a chance to heal. There are various methods used to deliver radiation therapy, including whole and partial-breast radiation. Partial breast radiation is considered the optimal treatment of most patients because a smaller part of the breast is irradiated. Although the dose is higher, the full course takes less time than whole breast irradiation. Both whole and partial breast radiation commonly result in skin burns of various depths.

Surgical Interventions

For those who present with earlier stages of breast cancer (I/II), resection of the mass is the initial step with the option of BCS (lumpectomy) or mastectomy with/without axillary lymph node dissection (ALND).[25] Lowest recurrence rates exist with Lumina A (HR-positive [estrogen/progesterone] and HER2-negative cancers.[25] If mastectomy is not chosen, BCS along with sentinel lymph node biopsy or ALND will be done, followed by radiation therapy.[14]

Breast-conserving surgery

BCS involves resecting the malignant mass with clear (negative) margins that will yield a cosmetically acceptable outcome. BCS is typically paired with subsequent breast irradiation.[25] There are multiple contraindications for BCS, including malignant or suspicious calcifications outside of the lesion, lesions that cannot be resected with negative margins and still result in a cosmetically acceptable result, and contraindications for subsequent radiation therapy.[25] Although patients with BRCA 1 or BRCA 2 mutations are not excluded from BCS consideration, bilateral mastectomy should be considered due to the increased likelihood of recurrence.[25] Despite the recommendations regarding BCS, some patients will opt for a mastectomy with or without reconstruction.

Mastectomy
Mastectomy, by definition, is the surgical removal of breast tissue. There are various mastectomy approaches available to patients based on the size and location of the mass and their reconstruction wishes. The more common mastectomies include total mastectomy, skin-sparing mastectomy, and nipple-sparing mastectomy.[25] Total mastectomy removes the entire breast parenchyma, nipple/areola, and much of the skin.[25] Skin-sparing mastectomy resembles total mastectomy except that much of the skin is remaining to facilitate reconstruction with an autologous flap or expander/implant.[25] Finally, the nipple/areolar-sparing procedure preserves the complex and the skin used in the reconstructive process.[25] The inclusion criteria vary, but overall, patients with tumors no larger than 3 cm and at least 1 cm from the nipple can be considered for the latter 2 mastectomy options.[25] Any of these mastectomy approaches may involve ALND.

Axillary lymph node dissection
ALND has long been considered the gold-standard approach to treating breast cancer.[26] There is more than a 25% risk of regional recurrence of breast cancer in patients with 4 or more positive axillary lymph nodes.[25] A self-limiting complication of ALND is axillary web syndrome in which fibrotic bands/cords develop. Although the symptoms of axillary pain radiating down the ipsilateral arm can contribute to significant discomfort and reduced shoulder mobility, most patients experience a spontaneous resolution beginning at 3 months postop up to 1 year following ALND. Pain management is vital until the complication has been resolved.[27]

Lymphedema occurs when there is a disruption to normal lymphatic flow, leading to edema of the ipsilateral arm and chest. Although it may occur with a sentinel node biopsy, it is a common complication on ALND in up to 30% of patients. Radiation is considered to contribute to the likelihood, which may be paroxysmal edema that resolves.[20] Numbness may occur following ALND secondary to disruption of the axillary intercostobrachial nerve that innervates the skin.[28]

Staging and Prognosis of Breast Cancer

Tumor-Node-Metastasis staging
Staging breast cancer is intricate and unique. For many years, the staging was based on local, regional (spread to nearby lymph node (LN)), and metastatic (spread to distant organs) disease, which led to the tumor-node-metastasis (TNM) system. Staging remains essential to allow providers to develop an evidence-based treatment approach, prognosis, and surveillance plans.[29] See **Table 3**.

The American Joint Committee on Cancer (AJCC) recently updated the staging system for breast cancer to include clinical and pathologic staging.[2] Clinical staging is used when surgery is not the initial intervention approach, using several clinical elements, including the examination findings, imaging, and biopsy. Pathologic staging is concurrent with surgical intervention and assessment of the mass by a pathologist.[30]

SEER database and prognosis
Surveillance, epidemiology, and end results (SEER), or the Surveillance, Epidemiology, and End Results Program, tracks 5-year relative survival rates (RSR) for US breast cancers.[31] The SEER RSR is based on how far cancer has spread.[31] RSR is the percentage of survivors of the effects of their cancers, based on large groups of patients.[32] The SEER database does not use the AJCC TNM staging groups but categorizes cancers into localized (no spread of cancer), regional (spread nearby or to lymph nodes), and distant (spread to distant organs).[31] In 2021, the SEER data

estimates 281,500 new breast cancer cases and 43,600 deaths. The 5-year RSR (2011–2017) is 90.3%, with an RSR of 99% in localized disease, 86% in regional disease, 29% in distant disease, and 58% in unknown.[32]

Breast Cancer Screening

Breast cancer screening recommendations are often confusing and conflicting because different stakeholders and professional organizations publish their own proprietary guidelines. However, some have overlapping consistencies, such as with the American College of Obstetrics and Gynecology (ACOG), the United States Preventive Services Task Force (USPSTF), and the National Comprehensive Cancer Network (NCCN).[33] ACOG and the NCCN currently recommend a woman to undergo a clinical breast examination every 1 to 3 years between the ages of 25 to 39 years, and annually once they turn 40 years. The USPSTF does not recommend clinical breast examinations in any patients.[33,34] The ACOG and NCCN recommend mammography screening be offered to women at age 40 years, whereas the USPSTF recommends it begin at age 50 years.[33,34] All 3 organizations agree that annual screening is appropriate, with the USPSTF caveat that biennial screening begins at 55 years.[33,34] After age 75, the ACOG supports no longer offering mammography screening. USPSTF and NCCN both recommend that mammography screening cease when life expectancy does not exceed 10 years.[33,34]

Breast Cancer Survivorship

The NCCN Guidelines Version 2.2020 defines survivorship based on the impact of diagnosis and treatment of cancer and the many affected areas for the patient and their family members.[35] Survivorship begins at diagnosis and includes ongoing treatment and clinical remission.[35] Life after cancer is a vital part of survivorship. Understanding the impact of breast cancer on a patient's physical and mental health is imperative. Treatments are often anxiety-provoking and may make patients very sick. Often patients are dealing with anxiety and depression as a result of breast cancer.

Lifestyle impact is significant in survivorship. Many patients embrace significant lifestyle changes resulting from breast cancer, such as dietary changes, exercise, and smoking cessation. The support of their provider is key to their success. Self-perceptions often change after a breast cancer diagnosis. When coupled with cognitive changes (chemo-brain) and induced menopause, patients may experience a significant negative impact on both their personal and professional perceptions. The side effect of breast cancer treatments can alter libido, and a change in body habitus may negatively affect the sexuality of survivors. Engaging in discussions about intimacy and sexuality while providing resources to help patients navigate this difficulty remains an essential survivorship element. Awareness of the financial impact of surviving breast cancer is imperative. Providers must consider the out-of-pocket healthcare-related expenses surrounding surgical interventions, chemotherapy and/or radiation, or medication costs. However, loss of work may equal loss of wages. Many patients with breast cancer may have to choose between paying for care or basic needs, such as food, gas, and rent.[36] Survivors may have chronic side effects that require treatment or care throughout their lifetime. The cumulative financial consequences can be crippling and must be regarded during survivorship.

Survivorship care should include surveillance for recurrent cancer and prevention of new cancers while monitoring for lingering negative diagnosis or treatment impacts on the psychosocial, physical, and immunologic well-being.[35] Surveillance care includes coordination and collaboration among all patient providers to assure the survivor's needs are fully met, from routine maintenance to preventive care to acute care needs that may arise. Survivorship is living with cancer, navigating through cancer, and moving beyond cancer. The ongoing support and partnership of providers in this journey will potentiate a positive experience for patients.

SUMMARY

Breast cancer diagnoses remain prevalent in the United States. Early-stage breast cancer has various treatment options available, whereas later-stage breast cancer has fewer intervention options, choosing between neoadjuvant systemic interventions or surgical interventions coupled with adjuvant therapies. In addition, providers across many specialties will likely offer care to patients with cancer and survivors. Understanding the journey from diagnosis to survivorship is imperative for the best practice of medicine and partnership with patients because they fight to survive and thrive.

CLINICS CARE POINTS

- Postmenopausal obesity is associated with an increased risk of hormone-receptor-positive breast cancer, whereas premenopausal obesity is associated with triple-negative breast cancer development.[3]

- The consumption of 2 to 3 alcoholic beverages daily is associated with a 20% greater chance of developing breast cancer than those who do not drink alcohol.[3]

- Ductal carcinoma in situ accounts for 1 in 5 new breast malignant diagnoses but has a very-high cure rate.

- Lobular carcinoma in situ is associated with an increased risk of breast cancer developing in the ipsilateral or contralateral breast, and its incidence is increasing rapidly.

- Invasive lobular carcinoma is more common in postmenopausal women, is most often hormonally mediated, producing estrogen/progesterone-positive, HER2-negative tumors, and more frequently occurs bilaterally than invasive ductal carcinoma.

- Approximately 30% of patients using an aromatase inhibitor (AI) experience AI-associated musculoskeletal syndrome with symptoms so severe, they discontinue AI therapy.

- Care of the breast cancer survivor requires a multidisciplinary approach so that each of the patient's postcancer issues can be addressed and risks mitigated.

DISCLOSURE

The authors have nothing to disclose.

REFERENCES

1. How common is breast cancer? | breast cancer statistics. Available at. https://www.cancer.org/cancer/breast-cancer/about/how-common-is-breast-cancer.html. Accessed Aug 9, 2021.
2. Gradishar WJ, Moran MS, Abraham J, et al. NCCN Guidelines® Insights: breast cancer, version 4.2021: featured updates to the NCCN guidelines. J Natl Compr Canc Netw 2021;19(5):484–93.
3. Breast cancer risk factors: age. breastcancer.org. 2020. Available at. https://www.breastcancer.org/risk/factors/age. Accessed Aug 21, 2021.
4. Sun Y-S, Zhao Z, Yang Z-N, et al. Risk factors and preventions of breast cancer. Int J Biol Sci 2017;13(11):1387–97.

5. Types of breast cancer | different breast cancer types. Available at. https://www.cancer.org/cancer/breast-cancer/about/types-of-breast-cancer.html.   Accessed Aug 9, 2021.

6. Definition of adenocarcinoma - NCI dictionary of cancer terms - national cancer institute. 2011. Available at. https://www.cancer.gov/publications/dictionaries/cancer-terms/def/adenocarcinoma. Accessed Aug 9, 2021.

7. Ductal carcinoma in situ (DCIS). Available at. https://www.cancer.org/cancer/breast-cancer/about/types-of-breast-cancer/dcis.html. Accessed Aug 18, 2021.

8. Peila R, Arthur R, Rohan TE. Risk factors for ductal carcinoma in situ of the breast in the UK Biobank cohort study. Cancer Epidemiol 2020;64:101648.

9. Waldman RA, Finch J, Grant-Kels JM, et al. Skin diseases of the breast and nipple: benign and malignant tumors. J Am Acad Dermatol 2019;80(6):1467–81.

10. Thomas M, Kelly ED, Abraham J, et al. Invasive lobular breast cancer: a review of pathogenesis, diagnosis, management, and future directions of early stage disease. Semin Oncol 2019;46(2):121–32.

11. Invasive breast cancer (IDC/ILC) | types of invasive breast carcinoma. Available at.   https://www.cancer.org/cancer/breast-cancer/about/types-of-breast-cancer/invasive-breast-cancer.html. Accessed Aug 24, 2021.

12. Angiosarcoma of the breast | breast angiosarcoma. Available at. https://www.cancer.org/cancer/breast-cancer/about/types-of-breast-cancer/angiosarcoma-of-the-breast.html. Accessed Aug 21, 2021.

13. FJP Bonito, Cerejeira D de A, Dahlstedt-Ferreira C, et al. Radiation-induced angiosarcoma of the breast: a review. Breast J 2020;26(3):458–63.

14. Oncotype DX: Genomic test to inform breast cancer treatment. Breastcancer.org. 2021.   Available   at.   https://www.breastcancer.org/symptoms/testing/types/oncotype_dx. Accessed August 22, 2021.

15. Meta-analysis of the cumulative risk of endometrial malignancy and systematic review of endometrial surveillance in extended tamoxifen therapy - fleming - 2018 - BJS (British Journal of Surgery) - Wiley Online Library. Accessed Jan 17, 2021. Available at: https://bjssjournals.onlinelibrary.wiley.com/doi/full/10.1002/bjs.10899.

16. Hormone therapy for breast cancer | American Cancer Society. Accessed Jan 18, 2021.   Available   at:https://www.cancer.org/cancer/breast-cancer/treatment/hormone-therapy-for-breast-cancer.html.

17. Hale MJ, Howell A, Dowsett M, et al. Tamoxifen related side effects and their impact on breast cancer incidence: A retrospective analysis of the randomised IBIS-I trial. Breast 2020;54:216–21.

18. Visvanathan K, Fabian CJ, Bantug E, et al. Use of endocrine therapy for breast cancer risk reduction: asco clinical practice guideline update. J Clin Oncol 2019;37(33):3152–65.

19. Viswanathan M, Reddy S, Berkman N, et al. Screening to prevent osteoporotic fractures: updated evidence report and systematic review for the US preventive services task force. JAMA 2018;319(24):2532.

20. Targeted drug therapy for breast cancer. Available at. https://www.cancer.org/cancer/breast-cancer/treatment/targeted-therapy-for-breast-cancer.html.   Accessed Jan 18, 2021.

21. Hansel TT, Kropshofer H, Singer T, et al. The safety and side effects of monoclonal antibodies. Nat Rev Drug Discov 2010;9(4):325–38.

22. Chemotherapy for breast cancer | American Cancer Society. Available at. https://www.cancer.org/cancer/breast-cancer/treatment/chemotherapy-for-breast-cancer.html. Accessed Jan 18, 2021.

23. Anthracycline chemotherapy agents. Available at. https://chemoth.com/types/anthracyclines. Accessed Jan 18, 2021.
24. McGowan JV, Chung R, Maulik A, et al. Anthracycline chemotherapy and cardiotoxicity. Cardiovasc Drugs Ther 2017;31(1):63–75.
25. Moo T-A, Sanford R, Dang C, et al. Overview of breast cancer therapy. PET Clin 2018;13(3):339–54.
26. Veronesi P, Corso GP. Standard and controversies in sentinel node in breast cancer patients. Breast J 2019;48(1):S53–6.
27. Dinas K, Kalder M, Zepiridis L, et al. Axillary web syndrome: incidence, pathogenesis, and management. Curr Probl Cancer 2019;43(6):100470.
28. Breast cancer in lymph nodes | lymph node surgery for breast cancer. Available at. https://www.cancer.org/cancer/breast-cancer/treatment/surgery-for-breast-cancer/lymph-node-surgery-for-breast-cancer.html. Accessed Aug 23, 2021.
29. Cserni G, Chmielik E, Cserni B, et al. The new TNM-based staging of breast cancer. Virchows Arch 2018;472(5):697–703.
30. Stages of breast cancer | understand breast cancer staging. Available at. https://www.cancer.org/cancer/breast-cancer/understanding-a-breast-cancer-diagnosis/stages-of-breast-cancer.html. Accessed Aug 24, 2021.
31. Survival rates for breast cancer. Available at. https://www.cancer.org/cancer/breast-cancer/understanding-a-breast-cancer-diagnosis/breast-cancer-survival-rates.html. Accessed Aug 24, 2021.
32. Cancer of the breast (female) - cancer stat facts. SEER. Available at. https://seer.cancer.gov/statfacts/html/breast.html. Accessed Aug 24, 2021.
33. Breast cancer risk assessment and screening in average-risk women. Available at. https://www.acog.org/en/clinical/clinical-guidance/practice-bulletin/articles/2017/07/breast-cancer-risk-assessment-and-screening-in-average-risk-women. Accessed Aug 24, 2021.
34. Recommendation: screening for breast cancer | united states preventive services taskforce. Available at. https://www.uspreventiveservicestaskforce.org/uspstf/draft-update-summary/breast-cancer-screening1. Accessed Aug 24, 2021.
35. Denlinger CS, Sanft T, Moslehi JJ, et al. NCCN guidelines insights: survivorship, version 2.2020: featured updates to the NCCN guidelines. J Natl Compr Canc Netw 2020;18(8):1016–23.
36. Help paying for living expenses. Breastcancer.org. 2018. Available at. https://www.breastcancer.org/tips/paying/living_expenses. Accessed August 24, 2021.

An Approach to Common Causes of Nonobstetric Gynecologic Pelvic Pain

Janelle Brown, MPAS, PA-C[a],*, Kimberly Weikel, MPAS, PA-C[b,1]

KEYWORDS

• Pain • Pelvis • Gynecologic • Nonobstetric • Dysmenorrhea

KEY POINTS

• Some of the most common causes of pelvic pain in patients with a uterus and ovaries include primary dysmenorrhea, endometriosis, pelvic inflammatory disease, functional ovarian cysts, ovarian torsion, leiomyomas, and adenomyosis.

• The prevalence of some of the causes of pelvic pain, such as endometriosis, primary dysmenorrhea, and adenomyosis, is likely much more than estimated because of the difficulty of diagnosing these conditions.

• Prompt diagnosis is essential for conditions such as pelvic inflammatory disease and ovarian torsion in order to initiate treatment to prevent harmful potential sequelae including infertility, necrosis, and chronic pelvic pain.

INTRODUCTION

Pelvic pain can be a frustrating chief complaint for both providers and patients. Prompt recognition and intervention help to alleviate the burden of this common clinical complaint. This article seeks to educate providers on how to identify, workup, diagnose, and treat common causes of nonobstetric gynecologic pelvic pain. Providers should keep in mind that not all pelvic pain is related to the reproductive organs. The most common nongynecologic causes of pelvic pain include irritable bowel syndrome, interstitial cystitis, pelvic floor muscle tenderness, and depression.[1] **Table 1** outlines the various differential diagnoses of pelvic pain.

Disclaimer: This article reviews pathologies related to the female pelvic anatomy; however, not all people with this anatomy identify as female. This article will be void of gendered terms, unless citing studies that refer directly to women. The authors wish to be inclusive and represent the diverse patient population that can experience pelvic pain.

[a] Baylor Scott and White Specialty Clinic, 200 Medical Parkway, Austin, TX 78738, USA;
[b] UCHealth Women's Care Clinic - Anshutz Medical Campus, 1635 Aurora Court, Anshutz Outpatient Pavilion, Aurora, CO 80045, USA
[1] Present address: 2538 Elm Street, Denver, CO 80207.
* Corresponding author. Baylor Scott and White Specialty Clinic, 200 Medical Parkway, Austin, TX 78738.
E-mail address: jebrown727@gmail.com

Physician Assist Clin 7 (2022) 447–463
https://doi.org/10.1016/j.cpha.2022.02.006
2405-7991/22/© 2022 Elsevier Inc. All rights reserved.
physicianassistant.theclinics.com

Table 1	
Differential diagnosis of gynecologic pelvic pain[2]	
Adnexal Causes	**Uterine Causes**
1. Ovarian cyst/s	1. Dysmenorrhea
2. Ovarian torsion	2. Leiomyoma (uterine fibroid)
3. Pelvic inflammatory disease	3. Endometriosis
4. Tubo-ovarian abscess	4. Adenomyosis
	5. Malpositioned intrauterine device

PRIMARY DYSMENORRHEA

Dysmenorrhea is defined as painful menstruation and is considered one of the most common causes of pelvic pain. Primary dysmenorrhea is defined as painful menstruation with no identifiable cause.[3,4] For reference, secondary dysmenorrhea is defined as painful menstruation with an identifiable cause and many of those causes (eg, endometriosis and adenomyosis) are addressed throughout this article. Despite the high prevalence, dysmenorrhea is often underreported and is therefore also under-treated. The disease burden of dysmenorrhea is vast, with many menstruating people having to miss work and/or school because of symptoms.[3] It is important that providers are able to address these concerns with their patients and formulate treatment plans to relieve symptomatology.

Prevalence

Primary dysmenorrhea commonly presents in patients 6 to 12 months after menarche but also has been reported to present up to 2 years after menarche.[3] It is estimated that dysmenorrhea affects 70% to 93% of adolescents.[4] Dysmenorrhea is reported as the most common cause of missing time in school. Approximately 20% to 40% of adolescents with dysmenorrhea report missing school, and 40% of these patients report that dysmenorrhea negatively impacts their ability to perform in school.[4] In addition, an estimated 600 million hours or $2 billion is lost in the United States annually because of missed work or reduced ability to function at work secondary to menstrual pain.[3] The risk factors for primary dysmenorrhea are outlined in **Box 1**. Typically, the severity of primary dysmenorrhea decreases as patients age and after childbirth.[3]

Pathophysiology

Painful menstruation is the result of uterine vasoconstriction and inflammation.[5] The most widely accepted description of the pathogenesis of primary dysmenorrhea is

Box 1
Risk factors for primary dysmenorrhea[3–5]
Age younger than 30 years
Menarche before 12 years old
Obesity or body mass index less than 20 kg/m^2
Cigarette smoking
Heavy and/or long duration of menstrual flow
History of sexual assault
Family history of dysmenorrhea

the overproduction of prostaglandins (PGs) and leukotrienes.[5] During the menstrual cycle, ovulatory progesterone levels stabilize cellular lysosomes. However, at the end of the luteal phase (ie, phase after ovulation and before start of bleeding) progesterone levels decline and the lysosomes break down and release an enzyme called phospholipase A2.[5] This enzyme triggers the cyclooxygenase pathway, which results in prostaglandin production. Prostaglandins are a group of lipid compounds that are involved in numerous physiologic and pathologic processes within the body, including regulating pain, body temperature, inflammation, and sleep.[5] There are 9 total classes of PGs. Specifically, class PGF2α and PGE2 are the major contributors to primary dysmenorrhea.[3,5] PGF2α causes uterine hypercontractility, which restricts blood flow, and it is also directly involved in arcuate vessel constriction.[5] Both uterine contraction and restriction of blood flow produce hypoxia that leads to the accumulation of anaerobic metabolites that subsequently stimulates pain receptors. Additional effects of PGs include headaches, nausea, bloating, vomiting, and diarrhea.[3–5]

Presentation

The most common symptoms of primary dysmenorrhea are listed in **Box 2**.

Diagnosis

Adolescent patients with a classic presentation of primary dysmenorrhea do not require an invasive physical examination or testing before starting empiric treatment. Transvaginal ultrasound (TVUS) or abdominal ultrasound is reserved for patients who fail first-line treatments or if a secondary cause of dysmenorrhea is suspected.[3] The physical examination should include vital signs, and it is important to record a blood pressure if oral contraceptives will be part of the treatment plan. An abdominal examination should be performed. A pelvic examination is not necessary but may be warranted if the patient is sexually active and an infection is suspected. With primary dysmenorrhea, the pelvic examination, if performed, will reveal a normal sized, mobile, and nontender uterus with the absence of mucopurulent discharge, uterosacral nodularity (seen in endometriosis), or adnexal mass.[3]

Treatment

The best treatment approach is for the provider and patient to partake in shared decision making so that the treatment plan will properly address the patient's individual

---

Box 2
Common symptoms of primary dysmenorrhea[3–5]

1. Symptoms presenting most commonly within 6 to 12 months of menarche and no later than 2 years after menarche

2. Pain begins right before menstruation and often lasts 24 to 48 hours

3. Pain does not commonly last more than 72 hours

4. Pain often at its worst on first or second day of menstruation

5. Pain is often episodic in nature and cramping can vary in severity

6. Pain located in the suprapubic region or lower abdomen and can radiate to the upper thighs and/or lower back

7. Symptoms are often similar with each cycle

8. Systemic symptoms can include nausea, vomiting, diarrhea, insomnia, and headache

needs and goals.[3] The first step in approaching primary dysmenorrhea is patient education. Patient education should include reviewing anatomy and pathophysiology of menstruation. Patient education also should include risks/benefits of pharmacologic and nonpharmacologic treatment options as well as addressing expectations. Using pictures or models is helpful for patients to be able to visualize anatomy. Recommending patients keep track of their menstrual flow and symptomatology will help them learn more about their bodies and can guide providers to tailor treatment plans. There are many free smartphone applications that can help patients accomplish this task.[3,4]

Nonhormonal treatment options

Nonsteroidal anti-inflammatories (NSAIDs) are the preferred first-line analgesics because they work by inhibiting the ultimate production of PGs.[3] Ibuprofen and naproxen are 2 examples of NSAIDs that can be found at a low cost and are well tolerated by most patients. Dosing can be titrated based on symptom control and toleration of side effects.[3,4] If patients can predict the onset of their menses, they should be counseled to start the NSAID 1 to 2 days prior. Other nonhormonal options that have varying efficacy but are relatively benign to try include the following: warm compress or heat, exercise, yoga, transcutaneous electrical nerve stimulation, and acupuncture.[3]

Hormonal treatment options

Hormonal options are especially appealing to patients who also desire contraception. Both combined hormonal contraception and progestin-only contraception can be considered.[3] Progestin-only options may be chosen as first-line if the patient has a history of deep venous thrombosis (DVT) or migraine with aura, which can be negatively affected by estrogen-containing options.[4]

Combined hormonal contraception options include pills, transdermal patches, and intravaginal rings. Progestin-only options include pills, intramuscular injections, and levonorgestrel intrauterine devices (LNG-IUDs). These methods work to decrease primary dysmenorrhea by inhibiting ovulation and decidualization of the endometrial lining, which will reduce prostaglandin and leukotriene production.[3,4]

ENDOMETRIOSIS

A difficult diagnosis to definitively establish, endometriosis is the most common single gynecologic diagnosis responsible for hospitalization of premenopausal patients.[6] Many cases never reach a definitive diagnosis because surgery is required for biopsy of endometrial implants. Thus, clinical suspicion is important to prompt initiation of workup and treatment for patients with presumed endometriosis.

Prevalence

Because diagnosis requires surgery, the exact prevalence is unknown; however, it is estimated to be present in 6% to 10% of reproductive-aged patients.[6] Access to medical care and ability to undergo surgical intervention are both limiting factors of establishing the exact prevalence.[7] Among women hospitalized for pelvic pain, the prevalence is thought to be between 5% and 21%.[7] Adolescents are an especially affected group, with endometriosis accounting for 49% of chronic pelvic pain cases and 75% of cases of pain that is unresponsive to medical treatment.[7]

Pathophysiology

The exact pathophysiology of endometriosis is unclear, but there are several leading theories. These include retrograde menstruation with transport of endometrial cells, metaplasia of coelomic epithelium, hematogenous or lymphatic spread, and altered immunity. Most cases are thought to likely be a combination of several of the theories. For instance, many likely have some degree of retrograde menstruation that is dependent on the capability of their immune system to eliminate.[6] There have also been descriptions of genetic components to the development of endometriosis, with studies demonstrating that 7% to 9% of patients' first-degree female relatives also being diagnosed with the disease.[6]

Presentation

The symptoms of endometriosis vary based on where within the peritoneum each patient has endometrial implants. The most common symptom of endometriosis is pelvic pain right before, during, and right after menstruation. Endometrial implants are most commonly found on the peritoneal surfaces of the ovaries, cul-de-sac, and bladder. However, lesions also can be found far from the pelvis in areas such as lung, joints, and even the brain.[6] Lesions may also develop in areas of prior incision, such as cesarean delivery scars. Another common presenting sign is infertility, with one-third of patients with endometriosis experiencing infertility.[7]

Along with signs and symptoms, the physical examination findings in patients with endometriosis are largely dependent on the extent of infiltration and the location of the endometrial implants. The classic description of a physical examination of endometriosis includes palpation of tender nodules in the posterior vaginal fornix, along with tenderness to palpation of the uterus. However, it is important to note that many patients with endometriosis will have an unremarkable physical examination. There are many seemingly vague physical examination findings that could be found due to endometriosis. Adnexal masses may be palpated because of the presence of endometrial cysts (endometriomas) on the ovaries. There may be implants visualized on the cervix or within healed incisions within the pelvis.[6] The uterus may be fixed secondary to adhesions.[6]

Diagnosis/Workup

The definitive diagnosis of endometriosis is established via surgical intervention by either laparoscopy or laparotomy with direct visualization and biopsy of the lesions. Before surgical intervention, ultrasonography may be helpful in visualizing endometriomas.[7] MRI also can be considered, which has a high sensitivity at detecting deep endometriosis.[7] There are no serum biomarkers that directly detect the presence of endometriosis. CA-125 may be elevated; however, its specificity is low. It may be useful after medical or surgical treatment for evaluation of recurrences.[6]

Treatment

In some cases, the clinician and the patient may choose to start treatment without a clear diagnosis because of the invasive nature of the definitive diagnosis. Treatment is driven by many variables, including the desire to preserve fertility, risk factors associated with surgery, the stage of the disease, cost, and medication side effects. The overall goals of treatment include pain control, preventing worsening of the extent of the endometriosis, and preserving or promoting fertility if indicated. The most widely used initial treatment option includes NSAIDs for analgesia, and hormonal medications such as combination oral contraceptive pills.[6] Other hormonal treatments include progestins via several routes, including orally, intramuscularly, and via an intrauterine device. Danazol (a 19-nortestosterone derivative with progestinlike effects), gonadotropin-releasing hormone (GnRH) agonists, and GnRH antagonists are among other options for medical treatment. All the aforementioned work by suppressing endometrial implants, and thus decreasing dysmenorrhea and pelvic pain associated with endometriosis.[6]

Surgical treatment typically involves laparoscopic destruction or removal of endometrial implants and adhesions.[7] Surgery is able to decrease pain in some but not all patients, and therefore clear expectations should be set before surgical intervention.[7] Hysterectomy with or without bilateral salpingo-oophorectomy also may be considered; however, among patients with presurgery pain, post-hysterectomy pain is 3 times as likely.[7]

Other treatment considerations include referral to other specialists, including pelvic floor physical therapists, psychologists, infertility specialists, and pain specialists.[7]

PELVIC INFLAMMATORY DISEASE

Pelvic inflammatory disease (PID) is an acute-onset condition that is infectious in nature and should prompt quick initiation of treatment. Treatment is aimed at treating the patient's acute pain, but should be quickly initiated to prevent potential harmful long-term sequelae, including infertility, chronic pelvic pain, and damage to other organs.[8] Scarring or destruction of the adnexa from salpingitis or a tubo-ovarian abscess (TOA) can lead to infertility, ectopic pregnancy, and chronic pelvic pain.

Prevalence

It is estimated that there are 95.5 million *Chlamydia trachomatis* and *Neisseria gonorrhoeae* infections each year, with 15% of those untreated cases leading to PID.[8] Although *C trachomatis* and *N gonorrhoeae* are the most common pathogens to cause PID, there are many other causative pathogens, which raises the prevalence of condition. One in 8 women with a history of PID have trouble becoming pregnant.[9]

Pathophysiology

PID is caused by the ascent of microorganisms from the cervix or vagina to the endometrium, fallopian tubes, and adjacent structures.[8] As previously mentioned, the sexually transmitted organisms *C trachomatis* and *N gonorrhoeae* are the most common causes of PID. PID also can be the consequence of polymicrobial infections involving microorganisms that comprise the vaginal flora (ie, *Gardnerella vaginalis*, *Haemophilus influenzae*, enteric gram-negative rods, and *Streptococcus agalactiae*).[10] Infection of the pelvic structures results in fibrinous or suppurative inflammatory changes, causing damage to the epithelial and peritoneal surface of the fallopian tubes and ovaries. This can lead to scarring, adhesions, and either partial or total blockage of the fallopian tubes, increasing the risk of tubal factor infertility and chronic pelvic pain.[8]

Presentation

Pelvic pain from PID is classically acute in onset and occurs during or shortly after menses. However, the symptoms and onset may be much more subtle.[8] The pain can be described as bilateral, pressurelike, and is often accompanied by back pain and purulent vaginal discharge.[10] Postcoital bleeding, dyspareunia, and dysuria also may be present.[8] More severe cases would include higher severity of pelvic pain, nausea, vomiting, and high fever.[10]

Speculum examination findings may include purulent vaginal/cervical discharge, cervical friability, and erythema of the vaginal and cervical tissue. There is typically cervical motion tenderness with bimanual examination, as well as tenderness to compression of the uterus and adnexal structures.[8]

Diagnosis/Workup

Diagnosis of PID should largely be made based on clinical suspicion. This is because testing in patients with PID may all come back negative/within normal limits, or may take several days to come back, which further delays treatment. Every patient suspected of having PID should be tested for *C trachomatis* and *N gonorrhoeae*. Endometrial biopsy showing histopathologic evidence of endometritis is the most specific test available, but is often not feasible in many clinical settings.[10] Laparoscopy showing evidence of salpingitis is also considered standard for the diagnosis, but again is typically not feasible.[8] Other less invasive tests may show nonspecific evidence of PID. For example, complete blood count may show leukocytosis with left shift and erythrocyte sedimentation rate and C-reactive protein may be elevated.[10]

If imaging is done, such as with TVUS or MRI, it may show thickened fallopian tubes, with or without free pelvic fluid. There also may be a tubo-ovarian complex seen, which could represent a TOA.[10] Ultrasound also can be helpful in differentiating PID from other nongynecologic etiologies, such as acute appendicitis.[10]

Treatment

Because of the potential harmful sequelae of PID, treatment should be initiated as soon as there is clinical suspicion for the condition. For initiation of treatment, it should first be determined whether or not the patient will require outpatient or inpatient treatment. Mild to moderate PID usually can be safely managed with outpatient treatment. Indications for inpatient treatment of PID include patients in whom surgical emergencies cannot be excluded (ie, acute appendicitis), pregnant patients, patients who have tried and failed outpatient treatment, patients with severe illness, and patients with a TOA.[10] The antibiotic treatment regimens for PID are described in **Table 2**.[10]

For inpatient treatment, parenteral agents can be discontinued after 24 hours of clinical improvement or after the patient has been afebrile for 24 to 48 hours, but

Table 2 Treatment of pelvic inflammatory disease[10]	
Outpatient Treatment	*Inpatient Treatment*
Ceftriaxone 250 mg IM in a single dose (or other parenteral third-generation cephalosporin) PLUS Doxycycline 100 mg PO twice a day for 14 d WITH OR WITHOUT Metronidazole 500 mg PO twice a day for 14 d	Cefotetan 2 g IV every 12 h OR cefoxitin 2 g IV every 6 h PLUS Doxycycline 100 mg PO or IV every 12 h
Alternative regimen:	*Alternative regimen:*
Cefoxitin 2 g IM in a single dose and probenecid 1 g PO in a single dose administered concurrently PLUS Doxycycline 100 mg PO twice a day for 14 d WITH OR WITHOUT Metronidazole 500 mg PO twice a day for 14 d	Clindamycin 900 mg IV every 8 h PLUS Gentamicin loading dose IV or IM (2 mg/ kg body weight) followed by a maintenance dose (1.5 mg/kg) every 8 h OR single daily dosing (3–5 mg/kg) *Alternative regimen:* Ampicillin/sulbactam 3 mg IV every 6 h PLUS Doxycycline 100 mg PO or IV every 12 h

Abbreviations: IM, intramuscular; IV, intravenous; PO, by mouth.

doxycycline should be continued to complete the full 14-day course. The decision to add metronidazole should be dependent on the presence of a TOA or if the infection is thought to be caused by anaerobic organisms, such as with bacterial vaginosis. Alternatively, clindamycin may be added in place of metronidazole.[10]

FUNCTIONAL OVARIAN CYSTS

The most common ovarian cysts include follicular cysts and corpus luteal cysts, which are more broadly defined as functional or physiologic cysts. Types of benign pathologic or nonfunctional adnexal cysts include paratubal/paraovarian cysts, endometriomas, benign cystic teratomas, or benign serous or mucinous cystadenomas. Types of ovarian borderline or malignant tumors include germ cell, granulosa cell, or epithelial tumors.[11] Small ovarian cysts (ie, <4.0 cm) on their own are often asymptomatic. However, they are likely to cause pelvic pain when they grow at a rapid rate, hemorrhage, rupture, or cause a torsion.[2,12]

Prevalence

Ovarian cysts can form at any age, but are most common in the reproductive-age group because of endogenous hormones.[12] It should be noted that cyst rupture is also more common within this age group. It is challenging to determine the exact prevalence of ovarian cysts because many patients are asymptomatic. Follicular and corpus luteal cysts are most common, with follicular cysts occurring more frequently than corpus luteal cysts.[11] Corpus luteal cysts are more likely to lead to hemorrhage or rupture.[2]

Pathophysiology

A follicular cyst forms when the nondominant follicle does not properly reabsorb and grows. Follicular cysts have thin, smooth walls, no vasculature, and are unilocular, meaning these cysts have no internal septa, papillary projections, or solid components. Corpus luteal cysts form from the corpus luteum after ovulation in the luteal phase of the menstrual cycle. Unlike follicular cysts, corpus luteal cysts have thick irregular walls and are hypervascular.[2]

The risk for rupture of an ovarian cyst increases with ovulation. Agents used to induce ovulation can increase the risk of cyst formation because of the stimulating effects to the ovary. Oral contraceptive pills (OCPs) reduce the risk of cyst formation.[2]

Presentation

Ovarian cysts that are <4 cm are often asymptomatic. Larger persistent ovarian cysts may cause chronic pressurelike pain that can be cyclical or noncyclical in nature. Ovarian cysts >5 cm also present a greater risk of ovarian torsion. Cystic rupture often presents with sudden-onset unilateral sharp to dull or sometimes colicky pain.[2] Pain can persist after rupture for days to weeks because of free fluid in the peritoneal cavity. Patients also may report discomfort with sexual intercourse.[2] For many patients, it can be difficult to discern if the pain originates from the pelvis or lower abdomen. For example, in the emergency department (ED), abdominal pain is the chief complaint of 5% to 10% of patients annually, and there are no specific data relaying the number of ED visits due to pelvic pain.[2]

Diagnosis/Workup

Physical examination should include an abdominal examination. A bimanual examination is helpful to determine the exact area of tenderness and to palpate an adnexal mass. A speculum examination may be appropriate if an infection is suspected or if the patient is reporting irregular bleeding. It should be noted that ovarian cysts <4 cm can be difficult to palpate with a bimanual examination.[13] A urine pregnancy or serum β-human chorionic gonadotropin (β-hCG) test is warranted in reproductive-age patients, as it can affect treatment options. The imaging modality of choice is TVUS, which can diagnose the presence of a cyst and/or free fluid in the peritoneal cavity.[13] TVUS is also used to characterize the cyst. **Fig. 1** provides an example of what an ovarian cyst looks like on ultrasound imaging. In cases of cyst rupture, the ovary may appear within normal limits, but the previous presence of a cyst is confirmed by free fluid in the peritoneal cavity.[2]

Treatment

Ovarian cysts that are not at risk of torsion or large hemorrhage can be managed conservatively on an outpatient basis with symptom management that includes pelvic rest, NSAIDs, and warm compresses. Most patients are referred to gynecology so that a follow-up TVUS can be performed in 4 to 6 weeks. Patients who are hemodynamically unstable because of large hemorrhage will need urgent referral to gynecology for evaluation and possible need for laparoscopy or monitoring in an inpatient setting.[2,12]

OVARIAN TORSION

Ovarian torsion is a rare cause of pelvic pain accounting for only 3% of all gynecologic emergencies and is the fifth most common gynecologic surgical emergency.[2] Although rare, the ability of the provider to promptly recognize ovarian torsion is essential to preserve ovarian function and fertility.[2,14]

Prevalence

As stated previously, ovarian torsion accounts for 3% of gynecologic emergencies.[2] Risk factors for ovarian torsion include a previous torsion, adnexal masses or cysts

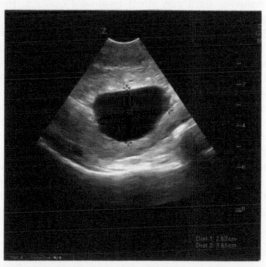

Fig. 1. A right ovarian cyst measuring 2.62 cm × 3.65 cm. Image attained via TVUS and represents a sagittal axis. (*From* Lee JY, Todd N, Truong J. Ultrasonographic and CT findings in ovarian torsion. *Visual journal of emergency medicine.* 2020;21:100869. https://doi.org/10.1016/j.visj.2020.100869; with permission.)

often larger than 5 cm, use of assisted reproductive technology (ART), which leads to hyperstimulation of the ovaries, polycystic ovarian syndrome, pregnancy, and previous tubal ligation. Benign physiologic cysts are more likely to cause a torsion. Conditions such as endometriosis, PID, and malignant lesions are less likely to cause torsion because they are often associated with affixing the ovary to the pelvic wall.[2,12]

Pathophysiology

Torsion can involve the adnexa, ovary, or less frequently the fallopian tube alone. Ovarian torsion occurs when the ovary makes one full turn around the infundibulopelvic ligament, also known as the suspensory ligament of the ovary, and the tubo-ovarian ligament along the long axis.[2,14] When torsion occurs, the venous system is impaired first, leading to stromal edema. Distal to the point of torsion, hemorrhagic infarction and necrosis of the adnexal structures occur.[14] Because the ovaries receive a dual blood supply from the ovarian and uterine arteries, it is possible to maintain perfusion despite torsion. As expected, the greater the number of rotations around the ligaments, the greater the degree of compromise to the vasculature. Torsion occurs less frequently on the left side because of the stabilizing effects of the sigmoid colon.[2,14,15]

Presentation

Patients with ovarian torsion usually present with unilateral severe sharp "stabbing" lower abdominal or pelvic pain that they characterize as intermittent and/or colicky.[2] Pain may radiate to the lower back and on abdominal examination rebound tenderness and guarding are often present. Nausea and vomiting are also frequently reported.[2,12]

Diagnosis/Workup

The ability of the clinician to promptly recognize ovarian torsion is essential to preserve ovarian function and fertility. A urine pregnancy or serum β-hCG test is warranted in reproductive-age patients, as it can affect treatment options. Pelvic ultrasound is the mainstay of diagnosis because it is readily available and does not expose the patient to radiation. Specifically, TVUS is the most accurate, and the sonographer should use the grayscale and color Doppler modalities to assess the torsion.[14] **Table 3** outlines the ultrasound findings consistent with torsion. **Fig. 2** shows an example of torsion seen on a TVUS. It should be noted that the persistence of arterial flow does not rule out adnexal torsion on ultrasound Doppler. Continued perfusion may be explained by the dual blood supply to the ovary from both the uterine and ovarian arteries or by intermittent and/or partial torsion.[14] MRI and computed tomography (CT) are other modalities that can be used to diagnose torsion. However, these modalities should not impede prompt initial ultrasonography if torsion is suspected. In the ED, a CT may have been the initial imaging modality used because the provider suspected a different cause of pain.[2] On CT, findings suggestive of ovarian torsion include deviation of the uterus to the affected side, adnexal enlargement, fluid in the peritoneal cavity (pelvic ascites), and deviation of adnexa to the contralateral side.[2,14]

Treatment

Ovarian torsion is a surgical emergency and should prompt immediate gynecologic consultation. If an ovary can be properly detorsed, there is an 80% rate of return to normal follicular development when follow-up postoperative ultrasound is performed.[16] If necrosis has occurred and there is no continued perfusion to the adnexal structures after detorsion, then a unilateral salpingo-oophorectomy is performed. In

Table 3
Ultrasound findings consistent with ovarian torsion[2,14]

Grayscale Findings	Color Doppler Findings
Increased size of ovary >4 cm	"Whirlpool sign" - twisted vascular pedicle
Hyperechoic stromal edema	Decreased venous flow
Peripherally displaced follicles	Decreased or absent arterial flow
Free fluid in peritoneal cavity (pelvic ascites) Twist of the ovarian pedicle "Follicular ring sign" - perifollicular edema	

addition, if a cyst was the cause of the torsion, then this is also addressed within the same procedure through drainage or removal of the cyst. To reduce the risk of retorsion, the surgeon may perform adnexal fixation.[2,16]

LEIOMYOMAS

Uterine leiomyomas, or fibroids, are benign neoplasms of the uterus that are commonly found by the age of menopause. Although often asymptomatic, leiomyomas will often cause abnormal uterine bleeding and also can be a cause of painful menses, noncyclic pelvic pain, and bulk symptoms.[17] Although bleeding symptoms are the most common symptoms associated with leiomyomas, the aspects associated with pain are highlighted in this article.

Prevalence

It is estimated that up to 70% of White people with a uterus and 80% of Black people with a uterus will develop uterine leiomyomas by menopause.[17] Just as they are more common among Black patients, they are also associated with more severe symptoms in this group.[17] The percentage of patients with leiomyomas is likely an underestimate, because many will go undetected because of being asymptomatic. It is thought that

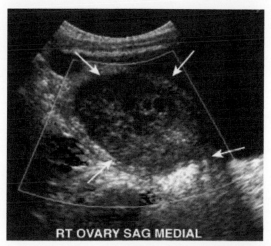

Fig. 2. An enlarged avascular ovary with multi-sized cysts consistent with torsion. (*From* Simpson W, Chaudhry H, Rosenberg HK. Pediatric Pelvic Sonography. In: *Diagnostic Ultrasound*. Elsevier; 2018:1870-1919; with permission.)

only 25% of patients with leiomyomas are symptomatic.[18] Increasing age up to menopause, nulliparity, early menarche, and initiation of oral contraceptives before age 16 are all risk factors for the development of fibroids.[17]

Pathophysiology

Leiomyomas arise from the alteration and replication of a single muscle cell within the uterine wall. The pathogenesis is poorly understood, but is thought to be multifactorial and regulated by hormonal and cytokine stimuli, epigenetic changes, and changes to the uterine environment.[19] Although risk is minimal, there is a small chance of myoma progression to leiomyosarcoma.[19]

Presentation

The symptoms associated with leiomyomas are largely dependent on the size and location of the fibroids within the uterus. **Fig. 3** displays the various locations and classifications of fibroids. Larger leiomyomas can lead to bulk symptoms, such as bowel and bladder dysfunction, including constipation and urinary frequency. Bulk symptoms also can include pelvic pressure and abdominopelvic protrusion.[18]

Risk of leiomyosarcoma also should be assessed when there is high clinical suspicion for the presence of leiomyomas. Risk factors associated with leiomyosarcoma include history of pelvic irradiation, use of tamoxifen, and rare genetic syndromes.[17]

Diagnosis/Workup

Uterine enlargement, with or without pain with palpation, is the key physical examination finding with leiomyomas.[18] Smaller leiomyomas located within the myometrium may not be appreciated on physical examination, thus further diagnostic evaluation should not be withheld if the physical examination is unremarkable.

TVUS is the imaging modality first used to assess the presence of leiomyomas.[18] Ultrasonography can also differentiate a leiomyomatous uterus from a gravid uterus or adnexal mass.[17] To determine the exact location and intracavitary extent of leiomyomas, saline may be infused into the endometrial cavity before ultrasound

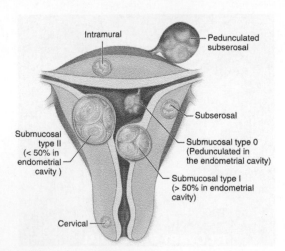

Fig. 3. The 5 types of uterine fibroids (eg, intramural, pedunculated, submucosal types I-II, subserosal, and cervical). (*From* Parikh S, Patel NR, Ferri F. Uterine Fibroids. In: *Ferri's Clinical Advisor 2022*. Philadelphia: Elsevier; 2021:1556-1558; with permission.)

examination.[17] This is known as a saline-infused sonogram (SIS). MRI with gadolinium contrast is an alternative imaging modality to SIS to better differentiate the location of leiomyomas, and also can establish whether a leiomyoma has devascularized or degenerated.[17]

Treatment

Considerations for treatment should be made based on extent of symptoms, age, menopause status, and desire for fertility. If the patient is asymptomatic, there is no evidence to support treatment.[17] Management options are either aimed at preventing blood loss alone, or preventing both blood loss and pelvic pain symptoms. Careful consideration should be made to ensure that the chosen treatment is aimed at treating the patients' primary complaint related to the leiomyoma(s).

NSAIDs are a reasonable initial treatment option.[17] GnRH agonists and antagonists, with or without concomitant therapy with low-dose estrogen with or without progestin, and aromatase inhibitors are medical agents approved for treatment of leiomyomas.[18,19] GnRH agonists, such as Leuprolide acetate, alleviate symptoms by inducing amenorrhea and by causing a significant reduction in uterine volume. These agents are indicated for short-term use (2–6 months) because of induction of bothersome menopausal symptoms and loss of bone mineral density.[17] The purpose of concomitant therapy with low-dose estrogen with or without progestin would be to mitigate these symptoms.[18] GnRH antagonists work by suppressing gonadotropins and ovarian sex hormones, leading to a reduction in heavy menstrual bleeding caused by leiomyomas.[17] Elagolix is a GnRH antagonist that when combined with estrogen and progestin (combination medication known as Oriahnn) is indicated for treatment of heavy menstrual bleeding associated with leiomyomas.[17] Similar to GnRH agonists, the addition of estrogen and progestin to elagolix is aimed at mitigating the bothersome menopausal symptoms caused by the drug.[17] Oriahnn is approved for use for up to 24 months.[17] Aromatase inhibitors, such as anastrozole and lotrozole, also cause a significant decrease in size (10%–70%) of uterine leiomyomas.[19] Like GnRH agonists, these agents also are indicated for short-term use only.[19] These therapy options may be considered in the months before surgical intervention with the purpose of reduction in size of the leiomyoma(s) or if the patient is nearing the average age of menopause.[17] There are other promising agents for treatment, such as selective progesterone receptor modulators, that are not yet approved in the United States.[19]

Surgical management options include either uterine-sparing options such as myomectomy and uterine artery embolization, or hysterectomy. Myomectomy can be offered to patients wishing to preserve fertility. This procedure can be done via laparotomy or laparoscopy, with or without power morcellation.[17] Regardless of the technique used, patients should be counseled that recurrence of leiomyomas after myomectomy is common, occurring in at least 25% of cases.[17] For patients who have completed childbearing or who do not wish to childbear, hysterectomy is a treatment option. Hysterectomy is the only treatment option that does not pose the risk of recurrence, which is common.[17] Uterine artery embolization (UAE) is a minimally invasive treatment option performed by interventional radiology that works by reducing the blood supply of the leiomyomas.[17] Pregnancy after UAE may be less safe than after myomectomy, and thus the patient's desire for pregnancy should be taken into consideration before choosing this treatment modality. UAE also has been associated with a higher prevalence of minor complications requiring additional surgical invention with hysterectomy.[17] Thus, if the patient is a poor surgical candidate, alternative treatment options should be considered.

ADENOMYOSIS

Adenomyosis is a benign gynecologic condition in which ectopic endometrial glands and stroma are pathologically found within the myometrium.[20] Adenomyosis can result in pelvic pain, abnormal uterine bleeding (AUB), dyspareunia, and infertility.[20] Up to one-third of patients with adenomyosis will be asymptomatic. Adenomyosis is abbreviated by the letter "A" in the acronym PALM-COIEN (polyp; adenomyosis; leiomyoma; malignancy and hyperplasia; coagulopathy; ovulatory dysfunction; endometrial; iatrogenic; and not yet classified).[21,22] This acronym is commonly used to classify AUB. There is no universally accepted classification of adenomyosis. However, within literature, clinicians may commonly see the classification system proposed by Grimbizis and colleagues in 2014. This system differentiates adenomyosis into 3 groups based on extent of disease: (1) focal, (2) diffuse, and (3) cystic adenomyosis.[21]

Prevalence

Before advancements in ultrasonography and MRI studies, the diagnosis of adenomyosis was made based on histologic findings after hysterectomy. Thankfully, advancements in imaging studies have aided in diagnosing this condition, especially in younger patients.[21] However, the exact prevalence of adenomyosis is difficult to determine because there are no standardized histologic or imaging criteria to diagnose it. One estimate based on ultrasound findings in the general population demonstrates a prevalence of 20.9%.[21] Risk factors for adenomyosis are listed in **Box 3**.

Pathophysiology

The pathophysiology of adenomyosis is not yet fully understood, and there are many theories. Some contributors to the disease include sex steroid hormone receptors, inflammatory molecules, extracellular matrix enzymes, growth factors, and neuroangiogenic factors.[20,21] One hypothesis is that the basalis endometrium is invaginated into the myometrium through an altered or interrupted junctional zone (JZ).[20] The ectopic endometrium is surrounded by hypertrophic and hyperplastic smooth muscle causing chronic peristaltic myometrial contractions that may induce continuous microtrauma and inflammation at the JZ.[20] Ectopic endometrial tissue can be diffusely disseminated within the myometrium or focal, most commonly occurring in the posterior uterine wall, forming a well-circumscribed area called an adenomyoma.[23]

Presentation

Symptoms of adenomyosis include dysmenorrhea, dyspareunia, and AUB.[20] Patients with symptomatic adenomyosis exhibit increased uterine contractility associated with dysmenorrhea.[20] Adenomyosis can cause heavy menstrual bleeding and is why it is included in the PALM-COEIN classification. Adenomyosis is also associated with subfertility and inhibiting successes with ART interventions.[22,24] There is some evidence

---

Box 3
Risk factors for adenomyosis[20–23]

Age older than 40 years

Multiparity

Previous cesarean delivery

Prior uterine surgery

Pregnancy termination

that adenomyosis often coexists with other benign gynecologic conditions, such as endometriosis and uterine leiomyomas.[21–23]

Diagnosis/Workup

Physical examination should include a bimanual examination, which may reveal a diffusely enlarged mobile uterus ± tenderness.[23] There are no laboratory tests specific to adenomyosis, but it is appropriate to order a β-hCG to rule out pregnancy and hemoglobin/hematocrit to assess for anemia if the patient reports heavy menstrual bleeding.

TVUS and MRI are the 2 imaging modalities used to make a noninvasive diagnosis of adenomyosis.[22] Hysteroscopy can also be used to assess the uterine cavity.[22] Although there have been many proposals for standard ways to diagnose adenomyosis based off of TVUS and MRI, more studies are needed to prove efficacy and come up with a shared classification system.[21] TVUS is the appropriate initial imaging study for patients reporting symptoms of adenomyosis. The sensitivity of TVUS to detect adenomyosis ranges from 65% to 81%.[21] Common imaging findings of adenomyosis are listed in **Box 4**.

Histologic evaluation of the uterus after hysterectomy is considered the gold standard for a definitive diagnosis of adenomyosis.[21,22] There is still debate on the depth of myometrial invasion necessary to make a diagnosis and this further emphasizes the need for a widely accepted set of diagnostic/pathologic criteria.[21] However, hysterectomy is not a viable option for all patients, especially those who wish to preserve fertility. For these patients, clinical suspicion along with TVUS and/or MRI findings are sufficient. Endometrial biopsy is not useful in the diagnosis of adenomyosis but may be appropriate in the workup of AUB if malignancy is suspected.[22]

Treatment

Treatment of adenomyosis is based on the patient's presenting symptoms, age, and family planning goals. NSAIDs should be recommended for pain relief. In patients wishing to preserve fertility and/or avoid surgical intervention, OCPs or an LNG-IUD are options mainly aimed to control bleeding patterns and dysmenorrhea.[21,22] Other medications, such as GnRH analogs, danazol, oral progestins, and aromatase inhibitors, have proven to be efficacious in limited studies.[21,22] More invasive interventions with the intent of maintaining fertility include cytoreductive and excisional surgery.[22] Procedures for patients not wishing to maintain fertility include endometrial ablation, UAE, and hysterectomy.[22] There is an emerging role of interventional radiology and high-intensity focused ultrasonography in the treatment of adenomyosis, but larger studies are needed to evaluate efficacy and outcomes.[21,22,25]

Box 4
Common imaging findings of adenomyosis[21,22]

Asymmetrical thickening of uterine walls

Intramyometrial cysts and/or hyperechoic islands

Fan-shaped shadowing of the myometrium

Myometrial echogenic subendometrial lines and buds

Translesional vascularity

Interrupted junctional zone (JZ) (the precise thickening of the JZ can be best measured on MRI and is often 8–12 mm)

CLINICS CARE POINTS

- When evaluating a patient with pelvic pain, providers should keep in mind that not all pelvic pain is related to the reproductive organs.

- As pelvic ultrasonography is commonly used to assess pelvic pain, it should be noted that the reliability of this imaging modality is vastly dependent on the experience level of the sonographer, as well as the interpretive skills of the radiologist. If clinical suspicion for a condition remains high after receiving ultrasound results, further evaluation should be pursued.

- Treatment of pelvic pain will largely depend on the menopausal status of the patient, as well as whether or not pregnancy is wanted.

- If pregnancy is wanted, providers can tailor treatment plans to the patient's goals for family planning. Treatment of pelvic pain is often multidisciplinary, with pelvic floor physical therapists, pain specialists, infertility specialists, and mental health providers often playing a crucial role, among others.

- When hormonal medications are chosen as the treatment for a cause of pelvic pain, a proper history is essential to ensure there are no contraindications to medication use, such as a history of seizures, DVTs, or migraine.

- Further research into adenomyosis and endometriosis is needed because both conditions do not have a clear pathogenesis and a definitive diagnosis can be made only after surgical intervention.

DISCLOSURE

The authors have nothing to disclose.

REFERENCES

1. Learman L, McHugh K. ACOG practice bulletin no. 218 chronic pelvic pain.
2. Dewey K, Wittrock C. Acute pelvic pain. Emerg Med Clin North Am 2019;37(2): 207–18.
3. Ferries-Rowe E, Corey E, Archer JS. Primary dysmenorrhea. Obstet Gynecol 2020;136(5):1047–58.
4. Sachedina A, Todd N. Dysmenorrhea, endometriosis and chronic pelvic pain in adolescents. J Clin Res Pediatr Endocrinol 2020;12(Suppl 1):7–17. https://www.ncbi.nlm.nih.gov/pmc/articles/PMC7053437/.
5. Iacovides S, Avidon I, Baker FC. What we know about primary dysmenorrhea today: a critical review. Hum Reprod Update 2015;21(6):762–78.
6. Ben-Meir A, Sarajari S. Chapter 58: endometriosis. In: Decherney A, Nathan L, Laufer N, et al, editors. Current diagnosis and treatment obstetrics and gynecology. 12th edition. USA: McGraw-Hill; 2019. p. 950–8.
7. Zondervan K, Becker CM, Missmer SA. Endometriosis. N Engl J Med 2020;382: 1244–56.
8. Brunham RC, Gottlieb SL, Paavonen J. Pelvic inflammatory disease. N Engl J Med 2015;372:2039–48.
9. Centers for Disease Control and Prevention. Pelvic inflammatory disease. Available at: https://www.cdc.gov/std/pid/. Accessed August 16, 2021.
10. Whiteley G. Chapter 45: sexually transmitted diseases and pelvic infections. In: Decherney A, Nathan L, Laufer N, et al, editors. Current diagnosis and treatment obstetrics and gynecology. 12th edition. USA: McGraw-Hill; 2019. p. 754–8.

11. Smorgick N, As-Sanie S. Pelvic pain in adolescents. Semin Reprod Med 2018; 36(2):116–22.
12. Malacarne DR, Ferrante KL, Brucker BM. Urologic and gynecologic sources of pelvic pain. Phys Med Rehabil Clin N Am 2017;28(3):571–88.
13. Speer LM, Mushkbar S, Erbele T. Chronic pelvic pain in women. Am Fam Physician 2016;93(5):380–7. Available at: https://www.aafp.org/afp/2016/0301/p380. html. Accessed 5 August 2021.
14. Ssi-Yan-Kai G, Rivain AL, Trichot C, et al. What every radiologist should know about adnexal torsion. Emerg Radiol 2018;25(1):51–9.
15. Melcer Y, Maymon R, Pekar-Zlotin M, et al. Does she have adnexal torsion? Prediction of adnexal torsion in reproductive age women. Arch Gynecol Obstet 2018; 297(3):685–90.
16. Huang C, Hong MK, Ding DC. A review of ovary torsion. Ci Ji Yi Xue Za Zhi 2017; 29(3):143–7.
17. Stewart E. Uterine fibroids. N Engl J Med 2015;372:1646–55.
18. American College of Obstetricians and Gynecologists. Practice Bulletin no. 228. Management of symptomatic uterine leiomyomas. 2021. Available at: https:// www.acog.org/clinical/clinical-guidance/practice-bulletin/articles/2021/06/ management-of-symptomatic-uterine-leiomyomas. Accessed August 14, 2021.
19. Dougherty M, DeCherney A. Chapter 42: benign disorders of the uterine corpus. In: Decherney A, Nathan L, Laufer N, et al, editors. Current diagnosis and treatment obstetrics and gynecology. 12th edition. McGraw-Hill; 2019. p. 675–80.
20. Vannuccini S, Tosti C, Carmona F, et al. Pathogenesis of adenomyosis: an update on molecular mechanisms. Reprod Biomed Online 2017;35(5):592–601.
21. Vannuccini S, Petraglia F. Recent advances in understanding and managing adenomyosis. F1000Res 2019;8:F1000. Faculty Rev-283. Published 2019 Mar 13.
22. Abbott JA. Adenomyosis and abnormal uterine bleeding (AUB-A)-pathogenesis, diagnosis, and management. Best Pract Res Clin Obstet Gynaecol 2017;40: 68–81.
23. Struble J, Reid S, Bedaiwy MA. Adenomyosis: a clinical review of a challenging gynecologic condition. J Minim Invasive Gynecol 2016;23(2):164–85.
24. Munro MG. Uterine polyps, adenomyosis, leiomyomas, and endometrial receptivity. Fertil Steril 2019;111(4):629–40.
25. Hai N, Hou Q, Ding X, et al. Ultrasound-guided transcervical radiofrequency ablation for symptomatic uterine adenomyosis. Br J Radiol 2017;90(1069): 20160119.

Behavioral Health in Obstetrics and Gynecology

Melissa Shaffron, DMSc, PA-C*, Elyse Watkins, DHSc, PA-C, DFAAPA, NCMP

KEYWORDS

- Behavioral health • OB/GYN • Depression • Anxiety • Mood disorders
- Postpartum depression • Postpartum psychosis • PTSD

KEY POINTS

- Women are at double the risk for developing a major depressive disorder than men in adolescence and extending through menopause.
- Mood disorders tend to wax and wane throughout the reproductive lifespan with a higher risk of relapse during pregnancy, postpartum, and the menopause transition.
- Postpartum depression occurs in 10% to 20% of the population, and screening for this disorder during the comprehensive postpartum visit is recommended.
- Symptoms of premenstrual syndrome can vary between mild and severe, and resolve when menstration begins.
- Patients with posttraumatic stress disorder need a multidisciplinary approach to treatment, including pharmacologic options and professional counseling.

Behavioral medicine diagnoses can be challenging and directly affect the quality of life of patients. These disorders can be exacerbated by hormonal changes during menstruation, pregnancy, postpartum, and perimenopause. Understanding the presentation and screening of all behavioral health disorders is imperative, as a delayed diagnosis can worsen the quality of life and negatively impact relationships. This article focuses on the most common mood disorders one is likely to encounter in general obstetrics/gynecology practice along with a brief mention of postpartum psychosis.

DEPRESSION

The pathophysiology and cause for major depressive disorder are not well understood and are likely a combination of genetic involvement and environmental factors. Genetic involvement has been noted in 30% to 40%[1,2] of patients diagnosed.

University of Lynchburg, School of PA Medicine, 1501 Lakeside Drive, Lynchburg, VA 24501, USA
* Corresponding author.
E-mail address: shaffron_mj@lynchburg.edu

Physician Assist Clin 7 (2022) 465–475
https://doi.org/10.1016/j.cpha.2022.02.002
2405-7991/22/© 2022 Elsevier Inc. All rights reserved.

Environmental factors that contribute to the pathophysiology of developing a major depressive disorder are increased stress, sexual abuse, trauma, and adverse childhood events. Major depressive disorder during pregnancy is associated with fetal growth effects, including low-birth-weight or small-for-gestational-age infants, and preterm delivery.[1,2]

The epidemiology of depression is well studied and documented. Major depressive disorder is twice as common in women as in men. During the lifespan of a woman, the risk for developing a major depressive disorder is equivalent to boys in adolescence and twice as prevalent in adolescence, which continues throughout the reproductive years until menopause. During and after menopause, the risk for female diagnosis of major depressive disorder equalizes with that of men,[1,3] but the menopause transition may exacerbate an underlying depressive disorder.

Patients may present with depression symptoms or major depressive disorder diagnosis already established. Patients may also describe a chief complaint of new-onset symptoms of feeling sad, depressed, or losing interest in activities they once enjoyed. New-onset symptoms should be clearly defined and documented. Common symptoms include the following[1,3]:

- Suicidal thoughts
- Loss of interest or pleasure (anhedonia)
- Feelings of guilt
- Decreased energy and fatigue
- Poor concentration
- Appetite changes
- Psychomotor agitation or retardation
- Sleep disturbances (insomnia or hypersomnia)

Adolescents with depression or major depressive disorder more frequently display symptoms of irritability than adults and less commonly report fatigue and insomnia. These symptoms may cause a lack of investment in sexually transmitted infection and pregnancy prevention. Weight changes in female adolescents can inappropriately be attributed to hormonal fluctuations or hormonal contraceptives, but they should always be addressed.[1,3] Excessive weight loss in an adolescent woman should trigger screening for an eating disorder.

Self-rating scales or clinician scales as screening tools can be used to help with the diagnosis of depression. Commonly used validated scales are the PHQ-9, PHQ-15, the Beck Depression Inventory, and the Zung Self-Rating Depression Scale. Medical evaluation to rule out other causes of symptoms is indicated for new or worsening symptoms.[4] The *Diagnostic and Statistical Manual of Mental Disorders* (Fifth Edition) (*DSM-5*) has set the following criteria for major depressive disorder[5]:

- Five or more of the following symptoms present for a minimum of two consecutive weeks and are a change from previous function. Must have a depressed mood, loss of interest, or loss of pleasure symptoms for diagnosis
  - Depressed mood
  - Diminished interest or pleasure in activities
  - Significant weight loss or weight gain or decrease or increase in appetite
  - Insomnia or hypersomnia
  - Psychomotor agitation or retardation
  - Fatigue or loss of energy
  - Feelings of worthlessness or excessive or inappropriate guilt
  - Diminished ability to think or concentrate, indecisiveness

  o Recurrent thoughts of death, recurrent suicidal ideation without a specific plan
    or a suicide attempt, or a specific plan for committing suicide
- Symptoms cause clinically significant distress or impairment in social, occupational, or other important areas of functioning
- The episode is not attributable to the physiologic effects of a substance or
  another medical condition

Treatment of depression and major depressive disorder should incorporate lifestyle changes. These can include exercise, smoking cessation, healthy sleeping habits, and relaxation training. Mindfulness-based meditation apps are readily available on smartphones. Psychotherapy can be used in conjunction with lifestyle changes to improve symptoms, allowing patients to cope with stressors and cognitive distortions. Various forms of psychotherapy are currently in practice, such as cognitive behavioral therapy, dialectical behavioral therapy, psychodynamic therapy, and humanistic/experiential therapy.

Pharmacotherapy is the mainstay treatment for depression and major depressive disorder and usually includes the use of selective serotonin reuptake inhibitors (SSRI) or serotonin-norepinephrine reuptake inhibitors (SNRI). Other pharmacologic options include atypical antidepressants, such as trazadone, and antipsychotics for severe depression. Each medication's symptom control, adverse effects, and prenatal effects must all be considered while prescribing (Table 1).[1,2] It is imperative to refer to psychiatry if a patient fails to respond to a trial of pharmacotherapy and psychotherapy, concern that the patient does not have a mood or anxiety disorder, experiences complications, or thoughts of self-harm.[1,2]

It is important to remember that patients with a history of major depressive disorder are likely to relapse during pregnancy and postpartum. Thus, it is essential to screen all pregnant patients during pregnancy and postpartum for depression and anxiety.

ANXIETY DISORDERS

Anxiety disorders include the diagnoses of panic disorder, social anxiety disorder, specific phobias, separation anxiety disorder, and generalized anxiety disorder.[5] Like most behavioral disorders, the cause of anxiety disorders is not well understood. Biogenetics, autonomic nervous system dysfunction, environmental stressors, and familial genetics are thought to play a role.[1]

Anxiety disorders have an overall 15% prevalence.[1,3] In adolescents, one in eight meets diagnostic criteria for an anxiety disorder.[1,3] Those diagnosed with an anxiety disorder are more likely to have other mental health disorders, substance abuse disorders, and physical health concerns. Generalized anxiety disorder affects 9% of the population across the lifetime with two-thirds of that population being women. Among anxiety disorders, generalized anxiety disorder is the most common. Panic disorder is twice as likely to be present in women, and Caucasians have a higher rate of diagnosis than blacks, Asian Americans, and Latinos/Hispanics.[1,3] This disparity may be due to implicit biases and cultural beliefs regarding mental health disorders.

Generalized anxiety disorder presents with persistent and excessive anxiety and worry. Patients have generalized anxiety, not limited to any one area of focus. Typically, worries are over items patients are unable to control and can result in interference with everyday life. Physical symptoms can include agitation, muscle tension, difficulty concentrating, and fatigue. Dysmenorrhea or chronic pelvic pain can also be physical symptoms present requiring consultation from women's health.[1,3]

Panic disorder is classified by the presence of panic attacks. Panic attacks present with an abrupt intense fear accompanied by physical symptoms. These attacks peak

Table 1
Commonly used pharmacotherapies for depression in obstetrics/gynecology[1]

Medication	Pregnancy/Lactation Effects
Citalopram	• No known teratogenicity • Possible risk of persistent newborn pulmonary hypertension and neonatal adaptation syndrome
Escitalopram	• No known teratogenicity • Possible risk of persistent newborn pulmonary hypertension and neonatal adaptation syndrome
Sertraline	• No known teratogenicity, low passage into breast milk • Possible risk of persistent newborn pulmonary hypertension and neonatal adaptation syndrome
Fluoxetine	• Considered safe in pregnancy • Well studied • Increased rates of neonatal adaptation syndrome compared with other SSRIs
Paroxetine	• A small increase in fetal cardiovascular defects • Possible risk of persistent newborn pulmonary hypertension and neonatal adaptation syndrome
Duloxetine	• Limited data • Increased risk of neonatal complications, especially when used during the third trimester
Venlafaxine	• Limited data • Decreased weight gain in breastfeeding infants
Desvenlafaxine	• Limited data • Should not be used if breastfeeding • Increased risk of neonatal complications, especially when used in the third trimester
Trazadone	• May have teratogenic effects • Risk of neonatal complications • Should not be used if breastfeeding
Bupropron	• Considered one of the safest antidepressants in pregnancy and lactation

within minutes and cause patients to change their behavior to prevent panic attacks. Physical manifestations can include diaphoresis, chest pain, shortness of breath, and palpitations.[1,3]

Self-rating scales or clinician scales as screening tools can be used for diagnosis. Some of the more commonly used validated screens are the Generalized Anxiety Disorder 7-item Scale or Beck Anxiety Inventory. The Edinburgh Postnatal Depression Scale-A is used specifically for perinatal anxiety. Medical evaluation to rule out other causes of symptoms is indicated for new or worsening symptoms.[2] DSM-5 criteria for generalized anxiety disorder include the following[5]:

- Excessive anxiety and worry, occurring more days than not for at least six months, about several events or activities
- The individual finds it difficult to control the worry
- The anxiety and worry are associated with three or more of the following:
  ○ Restlessness
  ○ Fatigue
  ○ Difficulty concentrating
  ○ Irritability

- o Muscle tension
- o Sleep disturbance
- The anxiety or physical symptom causes distress or impairment in areas of functioning
- Not attributable to effects of a substance or other medical condition
- Not better explained by another medical disorder

DSM-5 criteria for panic disorder include the following[5]:

- Presence of recurrent unexpected panic attacks during which four or more of the following occur:
  - o Palpitations
  - o Diaphoresis
  - o Shaking
  - o A sensation of shortness of breath
  - o Feeling of choking
  - o Chest pain
  - o Nausea
  - o Dizziness
  - o Chills or heat sensation
  - o Paresthesia
  - o Derealization or depersonalization
  - o Fear of losing control
  - o Fear of dying
- At least one of the panic attacks has been followed by one month of one or more of the following:
  - o Persistent worry about additional panic attacks
  - o Change in behavior related to the attacks
- Not attributable to effects of a substance or other medical condition
- Not better explained by another medical disorder

Treatment of anxiety disorders should include lifestyle changes. Additions that promote the improvement of the disorder and symptoms are exercise, smoking cessation, healthy sleeping habits, and relaxation training. Psychotherapeutic interventions include cognitive behavioral therapy, dialectical behavior therapy, exposure therapy, and psychodynamic therapy. These modalities can be used to learn coping skills, recognize triggers and cognitive distortions, and help to reduce anxious events. Psychotherapeutic modalities were found to be more effective when used with appropriate pharmacotherapy. Pharmacotherapy can include the use of SSRIs, SNRIs, and anxiolytic agents. These treatment options are the same as those utilized for the treatment of depression (Table 1).[1] Additional medications used in the treatment of anxiety disorders are listed in **Table 2**. Although the Food and Drug Administration changed the labeling of new drugs to exclude specific pregnancy categories, it is useful to list the previous categories of the most commonly used drugs concerning their potential adverse effects in pregnancy and lactation.

Benzodiazepines have been used for decades to treat anxiety disorders. As a drug class, they are classified as schedule IV of the US Controlled Substances Act. Thus, there is addiction and overdose potential. In addition, concomitant use of alcohol and/or opioids amplifies the risk of adverse events, including respiratory depression and death. Pregnant patients who take benzodiazepines are at increased risk of undergoing cesarean delivery, have low-birth-weight babies, and have newborns requiring the use of ventilatory interventions.[6]

Table 2	
Additional pharmacotherapy used for the treatment of anxiety disorders[1]	
Medication	**Prenatal/Lactation Effects**
Alprazolam	• Category D
Clonazepam	• Category D
Diazepam	• Category D; however, is indicated for the use in eclampsia
Lorazepam	• Category D; however, is indicated for the use in eclampsia
Temazepam	• Category X (should never be used in pregnancy) and avoid in breastfeeding
Estazolam	• Category X (should never be used in pregnancy) and avoid in breastfeeding
Flurazepam	• Category X (should never be used in pregnancy) and avoid in breastfeeding
Quazepam	• Category X (should never be used in pregnancy) and avoid in breastfeeding
Triazolam	• Category X (should never be used in pregnancy) and avoid in breastfeeding
Buspirone	• Limited data • Previously Category B
Gabapentin	• Significantly increased risk of preterm delivery and small for gestational age
Pregabalin	• Limited data, should avoid in pregnancy if possible
Quetiapine	• Category C • Associated with neonatal withdrawal symptoms

PREMENSTRUAL SYNDROME/PREMENSTRUAL DYSPHORIC DISORDER

The cause of premenstrual syndrome (PMS) is debated but is known to be linked to hormonal changes during the menstrual cycle. The prevalence rates vary for PMS with up to 80% of women experiencing PMS symptoms. Criteria met for the diagnosis of premenstrual dysphoric disorder (PMDD) are far less at less than 5%.[1]

Symptoms of PMS/PMDD will present one to two weeks before the next menstrual cycle and resolve once menstruation begins. The cyclic nature of the symptoms ties directly to the menstrual cycle. Symptoms can include depression, irritability, and anxiety along with physical symptoms of fluid retention, breast tenderness, and headache. These symptoms can be mild, moderate, or severe.[1]

History and physical examination alone can lead to a diagnosis of PMS or PMDD. Close monitoring of onset and improvement of symptoms in correlation with the menstrual cycle is most helpful. If symptoms are severe and negatively affecting the quality of life, a diagnosis of PMDD can be made.[1] The *DSM-5* criteria for PMDD include the following[5]:

- At least five symptoms present in the majority of menstrual cycles in the final week before the onset of menses and which start to improve after the onset of menses, becoming minimal or absent in the week after menses
- One or more of the following must be present:
  - Affective lability
  - Irritability or anger
  - Depressed mood
  - Anxiety

- One or more of the following (to reach a total of five needed, which can include symptoms listed above):
  - Decreased interest in usual activities
  - Difficulty concentrating
  - Lethargy
  - Change in appetite
  - Hypersomnia or insomnia
  - Sense of being overwhelmed or out of control
  - Physical symptoms present
- Symptoms causing interference with relationships or activities
- Not attributable to effects of a substance or other medical condition
- Not better explained by another medical disorder

Patients can track their moods with widely available smartphone apps or online platforms. Pharmacotherapy with SSRIs and SNRIs is effective in treating PMS and PMDD. However, it is essential to consider bipolar disorder in the differential because SSRIs can exacerbate bipolar disorder. Additional treatment with combined hormonal contraceptives has been shown to be effective. Supplements and herbal products are also used and can improve symptoms, but the evidence is weak. These alternative products include black cohosh, calcium 600 mg twice per day, chaste berry, evening primrose oil, ginkgo biloba, magnesium 400 mg/d, vitamin B6 (50–100 mg/d), or vitamin E (400 IU/d).[1]

POSTPARTUM DEPRESSION

The pathophysiology and cause of postpartum depression are not well understood and are likely a combination of hormonal changes and psychosocial factors. Associated impaired newborn bonding, infantile colic, breastfeeding challenges, suicide, and infanticide have been noted among patients who experience postpartum depression.[1] Postpartum depression occurs in 10% to 20%[1] of the general population. The risk of diagnosis increases with a previous diagnosis of postpartum depression, major depressive disorder, or bipolar disorder.[1]

When postpartum depression occurs, depressive symptoms begin in the first month postpartum in most patients; however, symptoms can occur during pregnancy and up to twelve months after delivery. Perinatal depression risk factors can include a history of depression, lack of support, domestic violence, nicotine use, and being in a lower-income socioeconomic category. Symptoms of postpartum depression include many of the symptoms experienced in major depressive disorder.[2,6]

The Edinburgh Postnatal Depression scale is the most frequently used screening tool in clinical practice. All postpartum patients should be screened during the comprehensive postpartum visit.[1,6] Postpartum depression *DSM-5* criteria include the following[5]:

- Five or more of the following symptoms present for a minimum of two consecutive weeks and are a change from previous function. (Must have depressed mood or loss of interest or pleasure symptom for diagnosis.)
  - Depressed mood
  - Diminished interest or pleasure in activities
  - Significant weight loss or weight gain or decrease or increase in appetite
  - Insomnia or hypersomnia
  - Psychomotor agitation or retardation
  - Fatigue or loss of energy
  - Feelings of worthlessness or excessive or inappropriate guilt

  ○ Diminished ability to think or concentrate, indecisiveness
  ○ Recurrent thoughts of death, recurrent suicidal ideation without a specific plan
    or a suicide attempt, or a specific plan for committing suicide
- Symptoms cause clinically significant distress or impairment in social, occupa-
  tional, or other important areas of functioning
- The episode is not attributable to the physiologic effects of a substance or
  another medical condition

Patients require emotional and educational support on the diagnosis and management of postpartum depression. Treatment with cognitive behavioral therapy and
pharmacotherapy is indicated. Pharmacotherapy treatment with SSRIs is preferred
with sertraline, venlafaxine, and fluvoxamine the most commonly used drugs.[1,7] Brexanolone is a gamma-aminobutyric acid-A receptor–positive modulator that is indicated for postpartum depression. It is an intravenous infusion over 60 hours and
can only be administered by health care providers and institutions that have been
certified in the proprietary risk and evaluation mitigation strategy. Patients require
continuous monitoring during the infusion. The cost of brexanolone is around
$38,000 per patient,[8] thus making it cost-prohibitive for most patients.

POSTPARTUM PSYCHOSIS

Postpartum psychosis is considered the most severe postpartum mood disorder,
affecting approximately 0.1% to 0.2% of postpartum patients.[9] Patients with postpartum psychosis may present with a range of symptoms, including mania, depression, confusion, anxiety, insomnia, disorganized thoughts, and hallucinations.
Postpartum psychosis usually occurs within the first four weeks following delivery
and is associated with an increased risk of infant abuse, neglect, and infanticide.[10]

History of bipolar disorder is the greatest risk factor of a patient developing postpartum
psychosis, as 20% of women with diagnosed bipolar disorder experience postpartum
psychosis or a manic episode.[11] Other risk factors include a family history of bipolar disorder, primiparity, and a history of a postpartum psychotic episode. A patient who is diagnosed with postpartum psychosis who does not have a mental health history is likely to
subsequently be diagnosed with bipolar disorder. Patients also have a 50% chance of
experiencing another mood disorder associated with pregnancy and childbirth.[12]

Specific DSM-5 diagnostic criteria for postpartum psychosis do not exist; rather, if a
patient experiences a psychotic episode within 4 weeks of childbirth, one can further
classify it by its relation to postpartum onset. Some mental health experts argue for an
increased timeframe after childbirth, possibly up to six or twelve months. When
assessing a patient for possible postpartum psychosis, the following information
should be gathered[13]:

- Is the patient sleeping, particularly when given the opportunity?
- Is this the patient's first psychotic episode?
- Is this the patient's first episode of postpartum psychosis?
- What is the patient's psychiatric history?
- Is there a history of illicit drug use?
- Is there a family history of bipolar disorder?
- Is the patient at risk of self-harm or harming others, particularly the child or
  children?

It is important to perform a complete physical examination, including a neurologic
examination. In addition, the following tests should be ordered[13]:

- Comprehensive metabolic panel
- Complete blood count
- Urinalysis
- Toxicology screen
- Prolactin (if Sheehan is suspected)
- Thyroid function tests
- Ammonia level

The differential diagnosis of postpartum psychosis[13] includes postpartum obsessive-compulsive disorder, postpartum depression, bipolar disorder, delirium, autoimmune encephalitis, Sheehan syndrome, drug intoxication, and medication reaction/interaction.

Postpartum psychosis is a medical emergency. Patients must be treated in the inpatient setting with psychiatric intervention. The pharmacologic management of postpartum psychosis includes the use of benzodiazepines, high-potency antipsychotics, and lithium.

POSTTRAUMATIC STRESS DISORDER

Posttraumatic stress disorder (PTSD) can occur following a life event that is considered beyond the typical or expected, such as intimate partner violence, sexual violence, natural disasters, wars/political conflicts, and violent deaths of friends or family. The epidemiology of PTSD varies according to the source, but approximately one in eleven people will be diagnosed, with more than half of those diagnoses in women.[14]

The DMS-5 criteria for PTSD[15] include the following:

Exposure to actual or threatened death, serious injury, or sexual violence in one or more of the following ways:

- Directly experiencing the traumatic event or event(s), witnessing the event as it occurred to others, or having a traumatic event occur in a family member or friend.
- Repeated exposure to details of the traumatic event or events.
- Intrusive symptoms associated with the traumatic event or events.
  - Recurrent and involuntary distressing memories of the traumatic event or events.
  - Recurrent distressing dreams in which the content and effect of the dream are related to the traumatic event or events. Note: In children, there may be frightening dreams without recognizable content
  - Flashbacks that feel as if the trauma was reoccurring
  - Psychological distress to cues that resemble an aspect of the trauma
  - Physiologic reactions to cues that resemble an aspect of the trauma
  - Persistent avoidance of experiences associated with the trauma
- Altered cognition and mood associated with the trauma
  - Inability to remember an important aspect of the traumatic event not due to a head injury or drug use
  - Persistent negative beliefs or expectations about self, others, and the world
  - Persistent blame of self or others
  - Persistent negative emotions, such as shame or guilt
  - Inability to feel positive emotions
  - Loss of interest or participation in activities
  - Detachment from others

- Hyperreactivity associated with the trauma
  - Irritability or aggression
  - Self-destructive/reckless behavior
  - Hypervigilance, including an exaggerated startle response
  - Difficulty concentrating
  - Sleep changes, such as insomnia, frequent nocturnal awakenings, and restless sleep not due to other organic causes
- Symptoms lasting more than 1 month and causing distress or impairment in personal, social, occupational, or other areas
- Symptoms not due to an underlying medical cause or substance

The treatment of PTSD usually involves a multidisciplinary approach with counselors, psychiatrists, behavioral medicine specialists, and even animal-assisted therapies. Cognitive behavioral therapies have been widely used for PTSD. The most commonly used pharmacologic agents are SSRIs and SNRIs, although their effectiveness has been challenged. Recent data strongly suggest that treatment with 3,4-methylenedioxymethamphetamine and a trained therapist show statistically and clinically significant effectiveness with a reduction in suicidality, little to no abuse potential, and no cardiac side effects.[16]

CLINICS CARE POINTS

- Patients with underlying mood disorders can experience exacerbations during major reproductive lifespan events, such as pregnancy, postpartum, and menopause.

- Some patients will present for the first time with a mood disorder during a reproductive lifespan event, such as pregnancy, postpartum, and menopause.

- Women should be regularly screened for mood disorders.

- Prompt diagnosis and treatment are recommended to avoid disruptions in the patient's life domains and mitigate adverse events, such as suicidality, infanticide, and work/interpersonal disruptions.

- The mainstays of treatment for most mood disorders are selective serotonin reuptake inhibitors and serotonin-norepinephrine reuptake inhibitors; the use of various counseling strategies can increase the effectiveness of these drugs.

- It is always important to consider the patient's plans for future pregnancies, as some medications are contraindicated or not advised for use in pregnancy.

DISCLOSURE

The authors have nothing to disclose.

REFERENCES

1. Osborne LM, Payne JL. Clinical updates in women's health care: mood and anxiety disorders. Obstet Gynecol 2017;16(5). https://doi.org/10.1097/AOG.0000000000002295.
2. Yonkers KA, Wisner KL, Stewart DE, et al. Management of depression during pregnancy: a report from the American Psychiatric Association and the American College of Obstetricians and Gynecologists. APA 2014. https://doi.org/10.1016/j.genhosppsych.2009.04.003.

3. ACOG Committee Opinion. Mental health disorders in adolescents. Obstet Gynecol 2017;130(1):e32–41.
4. ACOG Committee Opinion No. 757: screening for perinatal depression. Obstet Gynecol 2018;132(5):e208–12.
5. Diagnostic and statistical manual of mental disorders: DSM-5. 5th ed. APA; 2013. DSM-V. doi-org.db29.linccweb.org/10.1176/appi.
6. Yonkers KA, Gilstad-Hayden K, Forray A, et al. Association of panic disorder, generalized anxiety disorder, and benzodiazepine treatment during pregnancy with risk of adverse birth outcomes. JAMA Psychiatry 2017;74(11):1145–52.
7. ACOG Committee Opinion No. 757: screening for perinatal depression. Obstet Gynecol 2018;132(5):e208–12. PMID: 30629567.
8. Eldar-Lissai A, Cohen JT, Meltzer-Brody S, et al. Cost-effectiveness of brexanolone versus selective serotonin reuptake inhibitors for the treatment of postpartum depression in the United States. J Manag Care Spec Pharm 2020;26(5):627–38.
9. VanderKruik R, Barreix M, Chou D, et al. The global prevalence of postpartum psychosis: a systematic review. BMC Psychiatry 2017;17:1–9.
10. Perry A, Gordon-Smith K, Jones L, et al. Phenomenology, epidemiology and aetiology of postpartum psychosis: a review. Brain Sci 2021;11(1):47. https://doi.org/10.3390/brainsci11010047.
11. Wesseloo R, Kamperman AM, Munk-Olsen T, et al. Risk of postpartum relapse in bipolar disorder and postpartum psychosis: a systematic review and meta-analysis. Am J Psychiatry 2016;173:117–27.
12. Gilden J, Kamperman AM, Munk-Olsen T, et al. Long-term outcomes of postpartum psychosis: a systematic review and meta-analysis. J Clin Psychiatry 2020;81.
13. Osborne LM. Recognizing and managing postpartum psychosis: a clinical guide for obstetric providers. Obstet Gynecol Clin North Am 2018;45(3):455–68.
14. American Psychiatric Association. What is posttraumatic stress disorder?. 2020 Available at: https://www.psychiatry.org/patients-families/ptsd/what-is-ptsd. Accessed September 8, 2021.
15. American Psychiatric Association. Diagnostic and statistical manual of mental disorders. 5th ed. Arlington, VA: American Psychiatric Association; 2013.
16. Mitchell JM, Bogenschutz M, Lilienstein A, et al. MDMA-assisted therapy for severe PTSD: a randomized, double-blind, placebo-controlled phase 3 study. Nat Med 2021;27:1025–33.

Ovulation Induction in the Primary Gynecology Setting

Bianca Bae, MPAP, PA-C

KEYWORDS

• Anovulation • PCOS • Ovulation induction • Clomiphene citrate • Letrozole

KEY POINTS

- Clomiphene citrate (CC) and letrozole can be used for ovulation induction in the absence of other endocrine abnormalities, such as hypothyroidism and hyperprolactinemia.
- Ovulation induction medications involve increasing gonadotropin levels endogenously or exogenously. Use the lowest dose possible to induce ovulation. This may require some trial and error.
- The patient needs to have an intact hypothalamic-pituitary-ovarian axis to respond to CC and letrozole. Hypothalamic amenorrheic patients do not have an intact HPO axis, and therefore, should start off with gonadotropins.
- Limitations in the primary care setting include lack of access to in office ultrasonography and cost considerations with transvaginal ultrasound use.
- Referral to a reproductive endocrinology and infertility (REI) specialist is indicated if there is failure to conceive after 3 successful CC-induced ovulation cycles.
- Patients ≥ age 35 years and patients with known tubal or uterine pathologic condition should be referred to a REI specialist.

INTRODUCTION

Continuity of care is foundational in the primary care setting. It allows patients to gain confidence in their provider and providers to be better advocates for their patients. This patient-provider partnership is a special relationship that can facilitate early intervention that is more cost-effective and can be very advantageous in helping patients along their family-building journey. This is particularly true for patients living in rural and underserved communities, as access to care can be very limiting.

Infertility affects 1 out of 8 couples.[1] Although infertility workup and diagnosis have traditionally been managed by the reproductive endocrinology and infertility (REI) specialist, it is becoming more common for primary women's health providers to work up an infertility diagnosis and offer basic infertility treatment with ovulation induction (OI; **Table 1**). Safe, effective, and affordable access to infertility treatments is

There are no commercial or financial conflicts of interests.
Kindbody, PO Box 31787, Los Angeles, CA 90031-0649, USA
E-mail address: biancabae@alumni.usc.edu

Physician Assist Clin 7 (2022) 477–484
https://doi.org/10.1016/j.cpha.2022.02.007
2405-7991/22/© 2022 Elsevier Inc. All rights reserved.

Table 1
Ovulation induction treatment offered by primary women's health providers versus reproductive endocrinology and infertility specialist

	CC or Letrozole	Gonadotropins	TVUS	Trigger
Primary women's health provider	Yes	Rarely	Sometimes	Rarely
REI specialist	Yes	Yes	Yes	Yes

Adapted from FertilityIQ (https://www.fertilityiq.com/iui-or-artificial-insemination/the-biggest-decisions-in-an-iui-cycle#iui-at-a-fertility-clinic-vs-obgyn).

essential to combating reproductive health disparities, and physician assistants (PAs) can fill this gap when trained appropriately.

This article focuses on OI with timed intercourse as an initial treatment of ovulation dysfunction owing to polycystic ovarian syndrome (PCOS) and hypothalamic amenorrhea. Other less common causes, such as hyperprolactinemia and thyroid dysfunction, have their respective treatment modalities and are beyond the scope of this article. Patients diagnosed with unexplained infertility and age-related subfertility should be referred to an REI specialist to receive the appropriate counseling and treatment.

CAUSES/WORKUP

There are numerous causes for female infertility, including ovulation dysfunction, diminished ovarian reserve (DOR), tubal disease, and uterine factors. Ovulation dysfunction is the most common cause of female infertility, and PCOS is the most common cause of ovulation dysfunction in patients of reproductive age.

Amenorrhea and oligomenorrhea are clinical diagnoses. A thorough history of present illness and past medical history is essential when patients present with a desire to conceive but are having menstrual irregularities. Thus, menstrual history alone is sufficient and diagnostic.[2] The initial workup is done to determine the potential underlying cause. First-line laboratory tests include human chorionic gonadotropin (β-hCG), follicle stimulating hormone (FSH), estradiol (E2), thyroid stimulating hormone, prolactin, total testosterone, 17-hydroxyprogesterone, dehydroepiandrosterone, and hemoglobin A1c. Free testosterone, sex hormone binding globulin, and FSH:luteinizing hormone (LH) ratios are not necessary for a PCOS diagnosis, as they do not provide any information that would change the management of a patient seeking a conception.

History details, such as extreme exercise, extreme caloric restriction, and weight changes, in addition to physical examination findings consistent with hyperandrogenism and insulin resistance, can also help narrow the list of differential diagnoses.

OTHER WORKUP

Ovarian reserve is the amount of oocytes remaining in the ovary and is most reliably measured through an antral follicle count, performed through ultrasonography, and serum anti-Müllerian hormone (AMH). Days 2 to 4 E2/FSH have been phased out as initial markers for ovarian reserve, as AMH declines before FSH starts to increase.[3] Days 2 to 4 E2/FSH should be considered in patients found to have low AMH levels. A clomiphene citrate (CC) challenge test and serum Inhibin B are no longer considered the standard of care. It is important to note that ovarian reserve testing only provides information about oocyte quantity, not oocyte quality, and therefore, is not a predictor for spontaneous pregnancy. It can also provide valuable prognostic insight in a patient's response to ovarian stimulation, particularly when using gonadotropins, which is discussed later.

When there are comorbid male, uterine, or tubal factors, success rates of OI coupled with timed intercourse or intrauterine insemination (IUI) are very low. A semen analysis for the male partner should be done as part of the initial evaluation. Tubal patency can be confirmed with hysterosalpingogram, especially when a patient has risk factors, such as history of gonorrhea, chlamydia, pelvic inflammatory disease; history of any pelvic surgery; and endometriosis, as all of these risk factors increase the risk of adhesions. For a patient without these risk factors and under age 35 years, tubal evaluation may be deferred until failure to conceive after 3 to 6 treatment cycles.[4] Uterine cavity evaluation is done by saline sonogram, also known as saline infusion sonohysterography or saline sonohysterography. An abnormal saline sonogram may demonstrate endometrial polyps or submucosal fibroids distorting the uterine cavity, which will need further evaluation with a hysteroscopy before proceeding with treatment.

TREATMENT GOALS

There are different clinical indications for OI, and treatment should be individualized. Patients diagnosed with unexplained infertility or age-related subfertility may undergo OI, coupled with IUI, to promote multifollicular development in an effort to increase the chance of pregnancy. In contrast, treatment of oligo-or anovulatory women, including those with PCOS or hypothalamic amenorrhea, should be monofollicular development.

ORAL AGENTS
Clomiphene Citrate

CC is the most widely used oral agent for OI in a timed intercourse or IUI cycle. As a selective estrogen receptor modulator, CC blocks estrogen receptors at the hypothalamus, which stimulates gonadotropin-releasing hormone release and subsequently increases FSH from the anterior pituitary.[4] The elevated levels of FSH stimulates the ovaries and allows potential for multiple follicles to develop. Given this mechanism of action, a patient needs to have an intact, functioning hypothalamic-pituitary-ovarian (HPO) axis to respond to therapy.

Side Effects

Although CC is generally well tolerated, some side effects include mood swings and hot flashes.[4] It can also thin the endometrium and adversely affect the cervical mucus. Some rare but serious side effects involve visual disturbances, such as blurry vision, double vision, scotomata, and scintillations. Therapy should be discontinued if a patient reports visual side effects, as it can lead to permanent visual damage.

Clomiphene Citrate Regimen/Protocols

CC is administered orally and dosed starting from 50 mg for 5 days starting cycle day 2 to 5, following a spontaneous period, with a maximum daily dose of 150 mg.[5] Cycle day 1 is considered the first day of full flow. The dose is titrated up by 50-mg increments until ovulation occurs. The lowest dose needed to induce ovulation should be used.

A progestin-induced withdrawal bleed is not necessary to initiate CC in anovulatory patients. Data emerged demonstrating higher pregnancy and live birth rates following

CC use in anovulatory cycles compared with cycles where progestin-induced withdrawal bleeds occurred.[6] By not inducing a withdrawal bleed, patients' time to conception is faster.

Traditionally, when there is no evidence of ovulation or recruitment of a dominant follicle, the patient would wait for their next period or menses would be induced and a higher dose of CC would be administered at the subsequent cycle.

Alternatively, a "stair-step" protocol can be used, whereby a patient is immediately redosed up 50 mg for 5 days, with no need to wait for another menses. This approach demonstrated similar pregnancy rates but at a significantly shorter time to ovulation than the traditional protocol.[7] However, it is important to note that patients experienced more side effects with the stair-step approach.

Most patients will be pregnant within the first 3 to 6 cycles.[4] It is important to be mindful of potential long wait times to see the REI specialist. If pregnancy has not occurred by the sixth cycle, patients should be referred to an REI specialist to explore other options, such as in vitro fertilization. Advanced reproductive age (age ≥35 years) and increased duration of infertility are associated with treatment failure; therefore, these patients should receive timely referrals to see an REI specialist.

Letrozole

Letrozole is an aromatase inhibitor that blocks the production of estrogen by interfering with the androgen-to-estrogen conversion throughout the body, allowing an increase in FSH. It is commonly used to treat estrogen-receptor-positive breast cancer by decreasing circulating estrogen levels or inhibiting estrogen effects. Because of its mechanism of action, it emerged as an effective OI agent in patients with PCOS when a randomized control trial demonstrated that those treated with letrozole had a higher ovulation rate and almost a 50% higher live birth rate than those treated with CC.[8] Subsequent systematic review and meta-analysis supported these findings.[9] However, this is still considered off-label use.

Side Effects

Letrozole is better tolerated than CC, as it has a much shorter half-life. Common side effects include fatigue, dizziness, and hot flashes.

Letrozole Dosing/Protocols

Similarly to CC, letrozole is administered orally and dosed starting from 5 mg for 5 days starting cycle day 2 to 5, following a spontaneous period or progesterone-induced menses, with a maximum daily dose of 7.5 mg.[5] The "stair-step" protocol can also be used when there is no evidence of ovulation or recruitment of a dominant follicle by immediately redosing with an additional 2.5 mg of letrozole. **Fig. 1** provides a typical timeline.

INJECTABLES
Gonadotropins

Gonadotropins are subcutaneous injectable medications in the form of FSH or FSH/LH. Administering exogenous FSH directly stimulates the granulosa cells and promotes follicular growth. Gonadotropins should be used in conjunction with IUIs, not timed intercourse. Indications include failure to respond to CC and letrozole, DOR, and as initial treatment for patients ≥ age 40 years.

It is recommended to start off with a low dose of FSH, usually 37.5 to 75 IU/d and increasing in small increments after 7 days if there is no follicle greater than 10 mm has developed.[10]

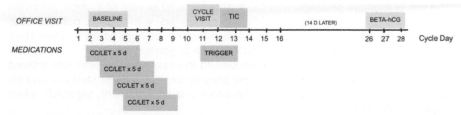

Fig. 1. Treatment timeline. (*Adapted from* FertilityIQ. (https://www.fertilityiq.com/iui-or-artificial-insemination/the-logistics-of-iui#natural-cycle-no-drugs).)

Hypothalamic amenorrheic patients benefit from exogenous FSH/LH administration, instead of exogenous FSH alone.[10] Patients with profound hypothalamic dysfunction should be counseled that duration of ovarian stimulation may be prolonged to achieve appropriate follicular growth. In addition, given the costs and risks associated with gonadotropin therapy, the American Society for Reproductive Medicine recommends only clinicians with the appropriate training and experience offer this treatment.[10]

Ovulation Triggers: Human Chorionic Gonadotropin

Physiologically, the LH surge allows for the final maturation of the egg and triggers ovulation. hCG is structurally similar to LH and is frequently used in OI cycles to precisely time intercourse or an IUI. There are 2 different types of commercially available hCG: urinary hCG or genetic recombinant hCG. The trigger injection can be 5000 to 10,000 IU of urinary hCG or 250 mg of recombinant hCG, which is equivalent to 6000 to 7000 IU urinary hCG.[10] Ovulation is expected to occur 36 to 48 hours after trigger. Patients are instructed to administer the hCG trigger when the lead follicle or follicles are 17 to 19 mm in diameter. Therefore, this medication can only be used in monitored OI cycles.

LUTEAL SUPPORT

Progesterone prepares the endometrium for pregnancy after ovulation by promoting secretory changes during the luteal phase. Exogenous progesterone is recommended in OI cycles using gonadotropins, not CC or letrozole.[11] Because gonadotropins directly stimulate the ovaries resulting in negative feedback to the pituitary and hypothalamus, normal corpus luteal function can be impaired. In contrast, CC and letrozole allow the body to maintain normal corpus luteal function.

COMPLICATIONS
Multiple Gestation

Multiple gestation is the most common complication from OI.[12] It is associated with increased risks to the fetus, such as prematurity and low birth weight, and to the mother, including gestational diabetes and preeclampsia.

Current Centers for Disease Control and Prevention birth data[13] indicate 3.29% of registered births in the United States were multiple pregnancies.[14] Of these births, 32.1 per 1000 live births were twin pregnancies and 87.7 per 100,000 live births were triplet or higher-order gestations.[14] Unfortunately, there is currently no national registry to help accurately determine what proportion of these births are due to complications of OI.

The risk of multiple gestation with CC is about 8%.[4] The rate of multiple gestation with letrozole is not significantly different compared with CC in patients with PCOS.[15] However, rates of multiple gestation can be as high as 36% when strict cancellation protocols are not placed with the use of gonadotropins.[10]

The goal is to use the lowest dose needed to increase the live birth rate without concurrently increasing the risk of multiple pregnancy. It is best to start low and increase the dosage as needed to allow monofollicular development, especially when using gonadotropins.

Ovarian Hyperstimulation Syndrome

Ovarian hyperstimulation syndrome (OHSS) is a rare but potentially life-threatening complication following ovarian stimulation, which involves ovarian enlargement, fluid retention, electrolyte imbalances, hemoconcentration, and hypercoagulability. Risk of OHSS is greater with gonadotropins than CC or letrozole. The risk of developing OHSS is higher for patients who have PCOS, are young, and have a low body mass index.[16] Signs and symptoms of OHSS include weight gain, bloating, shortness of breath, decreased urination, nausea, and vomiting. The treatment of OHSS is beyond the scope of this article.

BASELINE MONITORING

Patients should have a baseline ultrasound and β-hCG to confirm it is safe to proceed with therapy sometime during cycle days 2 to 5. The baseline ultrasound should always be done to rule out any ovarian cysts that may potentially be confused with follicular growth during ovarian stimulation. The β-hCG will confirm if the patient is pregnant. Obtaining a β-hCG level is a safeguard, as a miscarriage or ectopic pregnancy can be mistaken for a menstrual cycle. CC and letrozole are former Food and Drug Administration pregnancy category X and D, respectively.

IN-CYCLE MONITORING

Evidence of ovulation is essential in managing patients undergoing ovarian stimulation. This can be done with over-the-counter ovulation predictor kits (OPKs), transvaginal ultrasound (TVUS), and serum measurement of E2, LH, and progesterone.

Some primary care and OB/GYN clinics may not have in-office TVUS, limiting the options for monitoring to OPKs and serum hormone testing. Higher treatment costs owing to increased TVUS use are also a consideration when treating patients in the primary care setting. Over-the-counter OPKs are easily accessible yet can be cost-prohibitive for some patients. OPKs detect the LH surge, which precedes ovulation. Patients are advised to have intercourse the day of the positive OPK and the following day. Ovulation will occur 1 to 3 days after a positive OPK. Because sperm can last in the reproductive tract up to 5 days, whereas the egg is only viable for 24 hours, having sperm in the reproductive tract before the occurrence of ovulation is ideal.

Other monitoring options include basal body temperature (BBT) and serum progesterone. BBT tracking involves following the increase in BBT that naturally occurs after ovulation. A serum progesterone level greater than 3 ng/mL in the midluteal phase is consistent with ovulation. Therefore, these 2 methods are retrospective and not reliable in determining the timing of intercourse or IUI.

In contrast, patients managed in the REI setting are always monitored with serial ultrasounds and serum E2 levels (see **Table 1**) because these 2 modalities provide valuable information regarding a patient's response to the medication and informs treatment management.[10] This standard of care is based on the recommendation from Royal College of Obstetricians and Gynaecologists and National Institute for Clinical Excellence. Some have argued that TVUS is not essential in OI cycles; however, according to a systematic review, there is not enough evidence to reverse this recommendation.[17] TVUS allows for monitoring follicle recruitment, follicle size, and endometrial lining measurement. The information gleaned from TVUS allows for dose adjustments as necessary and determines timing of the trigger injection. In addition, serum E2 levels complement ultrasound findings. Approximately 200 pg/mL per mature follicle is expected.[5]

Patients taking CC or letrozole will return to the office after the 5-day course of medication to assess how the patient responded to the medication (see **Fig. 1**). Follicles grow approximately 1 to 2 mm daily during ovarian stimulation. If follicle size is not near 17 to 19 mm in diameter, the patient can be asked to return for a repeat ultrasound as needed. Of note, there is no utility in measuring serum E2 levels in patients taking letrozole because the E2 level will be significantly suppressed owing to the mechanism of action of the drug. Patients on gonadotropins will be seen more frequently for TVUS and bloodwork, and the timing will be based on the REI specialist's discretion.

PATIENT COUNSELING

If there are multiple follicles recruited, and there is a high chance of a multiple pregnancy, there should be a conversation to cancel the cycle. Cycle cancellation should be considered when the following occurs[18]:

- More than 2 follicles ≥16 mm
- ≥3 follicles measuring ≥10 mm
- Concern for developing OHSS

Patients should be counseled appropriately before initiating treatment regarding expectations and goals. The goal is to safely achieve ovulation that it is hoped results in a live birth, while minimizing the risk of complications and reducing side effects and costs. Patients should have a clear understanding of the indications for cycle cancellation, and providers should strictly follow these guidelines to avoid unnecessary and harmful sequelae.

CLINICS CARE POINTS

- A high anti-Müllerian hormone is not part of the diagnostic criteria for polycystic ovarian syndrome, and therefore, should not be used to diagnose polycystic ovarian syndrome.
- Always do a baseline ultrasound and β-human chorionic gonadotropin to confirm if is safe to proceed with therapy.
- Follicles grow approximately 1 to 2 mm daily during ovarian stimulation.

REFERENCES

1. RESOLVE: The National Infertility Association. How many people have infertility? RESOLVE: the National Infertility Association. 2018. Available at: https://resolve.org/how-many-people-have-infertility/. Accessed August 17, 2021.
2. ASRM. Diagnostic evaluation of the infertile female: a committee opinion. Fertil Steril 2015;103(6):e44–50.

3. Penzias A, Azziz R, Bendikson K, et al. Testing and interpreting measures of ovarian reserve: a committee opinion. Fertil Sterility 2020;114(6):1151–7.

4. ASRM. Use of clomiphene citrate in infertile women: a committee opinion. Fertil Steril 2013;100(2):341–8.

5. Ghadir S, Ambartsumyan G, DeCherney AH, et al. Chapter 53. Infertility. In: DeCherney AH, Nathan L, Laufer N, et al, editors. Current diagnosis & treatment: obstetrics & gynecology. 11 edition. McGraw Hill; 2013. Available at: https://obgyn-mhmedical-com.libproxy2.usc.edu/content.aspx?bookid=498&sectionid=41008657. Accessed August 22, 2021.

6. Diamond MP, Kruger M, Santoro N, et al. Endometrial shedding effect on conception and live birth in women with polycystic ovary syndrome. Obstet Gynecol 2012;119(5):902–8.

7. Jones T, Gualtieri M, Bruno-Gaston J, et al. Evaluation of clomiphene citrate stair-step protocol for ovulation induction. Fertil Sterility 2014;102(3):e138.

8. Legro RS, Brzyski RG, Diamond MP, et al. Letrozole versus clomiphene for infertility in the polycystic ovary syndrome. N Engl J Med 2014;371(2):119–29.

9. Roque M, Tostes ACI, Valle M, et al. Letrozole versus clomiphene citrate in polycystic ovary syndrome: systematic review and meta-analysis. Gynecol Endocrinol 2015;31(12):917–21.

10. ASRM. Use of exogenous gonadotropins for ovulation induction in anovulatory women: a committee opinion. Fertil Sterility 2020;113(1):66–70.

11. Green KA, Zolton JR, Schermerhorn SMV, et al. Progesterone luteal support after ovulation induction and intrauterine insemination: an updated systematic review and meta-analysis. Fertil Sterility 2017;107(4):924–33.e5.

12. ASRM. Multiple gestation associated with infertility therapy: an American Society for Reproductive Medicine Practice Committee opinion. Fertil Steril 2012;97(4):825–34.

13. Centers for Disease Control and Prevention. Multiple births. Multiple births. 2021. Available at: https://www.cdc.gov/nchs/fastats/multiple.htm. Accessed August 10, 2021.

14. Centers for Disease Control and Prevention. National Vital Statistics Reports Volume 70, Number 2, March 23 Births: Final Data for 2019. Published online 2019:51.

15. Franik S, Eltrop S, Kremer J, et al. Aromatase inhibitors (letrozole) for subfertility treatment in women with polycystic ovary syndrome. Cochrane Database Syst Rev 2018;5(5):CD010287.

16. Michalakis KG, DeCherney AH, Penzias AS, et al. Chapter 57. Assisted reproductive technologies: in vitro fertilization & related techniques. In: DeCherney AH, Nathan L, Laufer N, Roman AS, DeCherney AH, Nathan L, Laufer N, Roman AS, DeCherney Alan H, et al, editors. Current diagnosis & treatment: obstetrics & gynecology. 11th edition. McGraw Hill; 2013. Available at: https://obgyn-mhmedical-com.libproxy2.usc.edu/content.aspx?bookid=498&sectionid=41008661. Accessed August 22, 2021.

17. Galazis N, Zertalis M, Haoula Z, et al. Is ultrasound monitoring of the ovaries during ovulation induction by clomiphene citrate essential? A systematic review. J Obstet Gynaecol 2011;31(7):566–71.

18. Dickey RP. Strategies to reduce multiple pregnancies due to ovulation stimulation. Fertil Sterility 2009;91(1):1–17.

Pelvic Organ Prolapse

Christina Saldanha, PA-C, NCMP

KEYWORDS

- Pelvic organ prolapse • Female anatomy • Female aging • Menopause
- Postpartum • Pelvic floor physical therapy • Pessaries • POP-Q

KEY POINTS

- Pelvic organ prolapse (POP) is defined by The International Urogynecological Association and International Continence Society as the descent of one or more of the anterior vaginal wall, posterior vaginal wall, the uterus (cervix), or the apex of the vagina (vaginal vault or cuff scar after hysterectomy.
- POP is a clinical diagnosis, without the need for laboratory or imaging in most situations. Often times reported by the patient as a bulge in the vagina.
- A pessary is a first-line treatment of POP.
- Physical therapy and surgery are other options for treatment. After surgery, the recurrence rate of POP is 6% to 30%.

INTRODUCTION

Pelvic organ prolapse (POP) is a common problem many women may face throughout their life. POP is one of the most common reasons for a hysterectomy in the United States.[1] Although parity is the strongest risk factor for POP, there are many others including obesity, conditions that increase intra-abdominal pressure such as chronic cough, soft tissue abnormalities such as Ehlers–Danlos syndrome, family history, and age.[1–3] In 1907, Halban and Tandler came up with a hypothesis that injury to the levator muscle was the cause of POP and just recently this hypothesis was proven using 3D stress MRI, a study that was published in 2016.[4]

POP is a clinical diagnosis, without the need for laboratory or imaging in most situations. There are several ways POP can be treated, which range from expectant management, pessaries, pelvic floor muscle training (PFMT), and surgery. However, pessaries remain the first-line treatment of POP.[5]

DEFINITIONS
Pelvic Organ Prolapse

In 2010, the International Urogynecological Association (IUGA) and International Continence Society (ICS) released a joint report on the terminology for urogynecologic concerns including POP. They concluded that POP is "defined as the descent of one

PA, 3331 Healy Drive Unit 24067, Winston Salem, NC 27114, USA
E-mail address: camelcitywomenswellness@gmail.com

Physician Assist Clin 7 (2022) 485–497
https://doi.org/10.1016/j.cpha.2022.03.003
2405-7991/22/© 2022 Elsevier Inc. All rights reserved.

or more of the anterior vaginal wall, posterior vaginal wall, the uterus (cervix), or the apex of the vagina (vaginal vault or cuff scar after hysterectomy."[6] Important to note that this decent should correlate with the physical examination, and the clinician should try to avoid using the terms cystocele and rectocele because the exact organ that is involved with the prolapse may not be discernible from a physical examination alone.[7]

Pelvic Organ Prolapse Quantification

The IUGA and ICS have described the Pelvic Organ Prolapse Quantification (POP-Q) system that clinicians and researchers can use in practice. This system is the only validated method for objective measurement of POP, and it is useful when the woman may be going from clinician to clinician or to measure treatment success (preoperative and postoperative or pre-PFMT and post-PFMT).[6–8] The POP-Q system defines 6 points in the vagina: Aa and Ba are for the anterior vagina, Ap and Bp for the posterior vagina, and C and D for the cervix or vault. If she has had a hysterectomy, point D is not used.[8] POP can furthermore be divided into stages 0–IV, of which stage 0 is no prolapse, and stage IV is complete eversion of the vagina (**Table 1**). The hymen is the point of reference for prolapse description.[6] Again, the terms cystocele and rectocele are not used in the POP-Q or the staging system.

BACKGROUND
Anatomy

Because POP is a condition in which the normal anatomic state is compromised, it is prudent to understand the anatomy and how it influences this disease state. The levator ani muscle is the structural support of the pelvis in women, and when the muscle group is damaged, POP may be a consequence. There are 3 parts of the levator ani muscle: the iliococcygeal portion, the pubococcygeus portion, and the puborectal portion (**Fig. 1**). The iliococcygeal portion spans the space between both lateral sidewalls. The pubococcygeus portion inserts into the perineal body (the puboperineus

Table 1
Stages of POP. This is devised from the POP-Q system

Stage 0	No prolapse	No symptoms
Stage I	Most distal portion of the prolapse is more than 1 cm above the level of the hymen	May or may not have symptoms of prolapse
Stage II	Most distal portion of the prolapse is 1 cm or less proximal to or distal to the plane of the hymen	
Stage III	The most distal portion of the prolapse is more than 1 cm below the plan of the hymen	Very likely to have symptoms of prolapse
Stage IV	Complete eversion of the total length of the lower genital tract is demonstrated	

Of note, the point of reference is the hymen. Patients may have stage I or II prolapse on examination, but may not be symptomatic from this and therefore should not be diagnosed with POP. Diagnosis should largely be driven by symptoms, with the examination to support.

Data from Haylen BT, de Ridder D, Freeman RM, et al.; International Urogynecological Association; International Continence Society. An International Urogynecological Association (IUGA)/International Continence Society (ICS) joint report on the terminology for female pelvic floor dysfunction. Neuroural Urodyn. 2010;29(1):4-20.

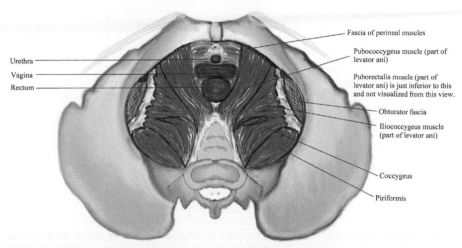

Urethra ——
Vagina ——
Rectum ——

Fascia of perineal muscles

Pubococcygeus muscle (part of levator ani)

Puborectalis muscle (part of levator ani) is just inferior to this and not visualized from this view.

Obturator fascia

Iliococcygeus muscle (part of levator ani)

Coccygeus

Piriformis

Fig. 1. Pelvic floor anatomy in women. There are 3 parts of the levator ani muscle: the ilio-coccygeal portion, the pubococcygeus portion, and the puborectal portion. Puborectal portion is not pictured here because it is inferior to the pubococcygeus in this view. The urogenital hiatus is the opening in the levator ani in which the urethra and the vagina pass, and this is the area implicated in POP. (Original illustration completed for this article by K. Glen Saldanha, PT, DPT, OCS, TPS.)

subdivision), the vaginal wall (the pubovaginalis subdivision), and the anal canal (the puboanalis subdivision).[9] Coccygeus is not part of the levator ani muscle group, but it is part of the pelvic floor, and it is the most posterior muscle. Other important support structures include the endopelvic fascia. This is a dense, fibrous connective tissue layer. It connects to the vagina and bilaterally to the pelvic sidewalls, and it merges with the levator ani muscles. The muscles and this fascia all together make up the pelvic diaphragm (**Fig. 2**).[9] Another relevant anatomic landmark to discuss is the urogenital hiatus. This is the opening in the levator ani muscle in which the vagina and urethra pass. Furthermore, this is the area that a baby passes through as well as the area in which prolapse occurs. When the urogenital hiatus increases, so do the likelihood of organ prolapse. In normal anatomy, the levator ani muscle is constantly contracted, which keeps the genital hiatus closed. The most common cause of injury to the levator ani muscle is vaginal delivery, and models have shown that the second stage of labor puts stretch ratios of up to 3.3 on this muscle group.[9] One last important support structure to mention is the ligaments. These include the apical ligaments, cardinal ligaments, and uterosacral ligaments. The primary role of these ligaments is to stretch and tense to keep the pelvic organs mobile; they are not very good support structures. Some research shows these ligaments can have a change in their protein expression and thus increase the load bearing of the ligaments.[10] All levels of support are connected through the endopelvic fascia, which is continuous throughout the entire pelvic floor.[11] The motor nerves that innervate this area are S2–S4.[7]

Cause

The pelvic floor anatomy can be quite complex, and one of the glaring questions among anatomists has been which produces the most support: muscle or connective tissue? It has been found that 34% to 55% of women with POP have an injury of the levator ani muscle that results in more than half of the muscle bulk being damaged.[4]

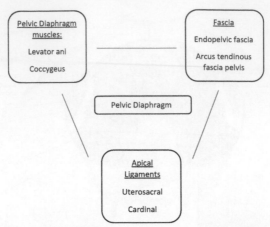

Fig. 2. The Pelvic Floor and interrelated support structures. The key anatomic structure for support is the levator ani muscle group. The fascia and apical ligaments provide secondary and tertiary support. All of this together makes up the pelvic diaphragm.

Because of this finding, it is believed that the ligaments and fascia play a minor role in support. After all, the levator ani muscle stays contracted for the most part, which keeps the genital hiatus closed. When there is damage to the levator ani (either the muscles themselves or the motor neurons that innervate this area), the support lies on the fascia and ligaments. Over time, this constant load will cause an irreversible stretch of the ligaments that will ultimately fail and result in prolapse.[3,9]

Risk Factors

The strongest risk factor for POP is parity. Women with one child show a 4-fold increase in the incidence of POP compared with the general population.[3] Other risk factors include increasing age, obesity, connective tissue disorders, such as Ehlers–Danlos syndrome, and genetics. Women with a family history significant for POP have a 2.5-fold increase of POP compared with the general population.[3] Instrumentation during vaginal delivery may also influence the risk for POP if any part of the levator ani is damaged. Defects in the levator ani muscle with forceps delivery are seen in up to 53% of women compared with 28% of women who did not have forceps-assisted delivery.[12] Also, because the levator ani attaches to the perineal body, and if the perineal body is damaged during childbirth, from an episiotomy, for example, this can contribute significantly to POP as well.[9] Obesity, along with other conditions that increase intra-abdominal pressure such as chronic cough, puts pressure on the pelvic floor weakening these structures, which increase the occurrence of POP by 40% to 75%.[1] Studies have shown mixed consensus whether chronic constipation or hysterectomy contributes to POP.[1,7,11]

DISCUSSION
Epidemiology

POP when defined as symptoms has a prevalence of 3% to 6% in the general women population and up to 50% when based on the physical examination.[13,14] Because clinicians will sometimes diagnose POP based on a physical examination alone, one may see values in the literature that suggest a prevalence of 3% to 50%. The average age women present to a provider care provider with symptoms of POP is 61 years, and prolapse of the anterior compartment is the most common followed by posterior prolapse and apical prolapse.[3] Prevalence has not changed during the last 10 years, and we expect that it may increase as the population ages.[15]

History and Physical Examination

The most likely presenting symptom patients may report is the sensation of a bulge in the vagina. Most women feel symptoms of POP when the leading age of the prolapsing area reaches 0.5 cm distal to the hymenal ring. For this reason, clinicians should use the hymen as the threshold because this can be standardized from clinician to clinician.[6,7,13] The most straightforward way to screen for POP is by asking women if they see or feel a bulge in the vagina. Women may also present with a discharge or bleeding if prolapsed tissue becomes irritated from rubbing on the inner thighs or clothes.[16]

Questions to ask during the history of present illness[6,7,16]:

- Does the patient see or feel a bulge in the vagina?
- Does the patient feel pelvic pressure or backache? Sometimes, this is described as period-like cramping.
- Does the patient have an unusual discharge?
- Assess bladder function by asking about frequency, urgency, stress incontinence symptoms, dysuria.
- Assess bowel function to understand if there is a history of constipation, straining, or digitation where the patient must use manual pressure to complete defecation.
- Is the prolapse causing problems during the patients' recreation or occupation?
- Is the prolapse causing symptoms of dyspareunia, coital incontinence, or sexual dysfunction in any form?

Of important note, mild descent of the pelvic organs is common and should not be considered pathologic. Thus, clinicians should base the diagnosis on symptoms with support from the examination.[7]

After the careful history is taken, an examination should be performed with the bladder empty.[6] Examination should include a speculum examination for visualization and a bimanual examination to palpate for intraabdominal masses that may be causing her symptoms. A speculum examination should also be done with a split speculum, where only one blade is used. This will help give visualization as to anterior, posterior, apical prolapse, and can be used with pressure against the posterior vaginal wall and then flipped around to apply pressure to the anterior vaginal wall. The patient should perform the Valsalva maneuver to give the clinician visual aid as to what is prolapsing. The perineum should not show any downward motion.[6] The examination also should be performed in the standing position particularly if the prolapse is not appreciated while the patient is supine.[6,7] POP-Q should be used to objectify prolapse both before, during, and after treatments.

Muscle testing can be performed at the time of pelvic examination simply via circumferential digital palpation and described qualitatively by using the terminologies: strong, normal, weak, and absent.[6,17] It is reasonable to obtain laboratories as necessary to rule out vaginitis or cystitis, but otherwise, laboratories are typically not indicated. However, clinicians should consider urodynamic testing in women who are considering surgical intervention as POP may mask stress urinary incontinence.[7]

Considerations on Body Image and Sexual Health

Clinicians should inquire about distress surrounding body image or sexual function in addition to the bothersome symptoms such as vaginal bulge, voiding symptoms, or defecation symptoms caused by POP. There are several validated questionnaires to help clinicians and patients understand their level of distress, 2 of which are the Pelvic Floor Distress Inventory (PFDI-20) and Pelvic Floor Impact Questionnaires (PFIQ-7).[18] These questionnaires look at 3 domains: urinary distress inventory, POP distress inventory, and colorectal-anal distress inventory. It is reasonable to consider using 1 of these questionnaires in clinical practice if the clinician is wanting to get a better understanding of how POP may be affecting the patient's life, particularly in risk, benefit, and alternative discussion about treatment options. People with POP are more likely to think self-conscious about their body, think less physically attractive, think less feminine, and think less sexually attractive.[19] POP affects the sexual organs, so it is prudent to consider the effect of POP on women's sexual health. Sexual health can be defined by the World Health Organization as "a state of physical, emotional, mental and social well-being in relation to sexuality; it is not merely the absence of disease."[20] Furthermore, sexual dysfunction is one of the more common presenting problems to a health care provider, and it is wise to consider screening for POP. Women with POP are more likely to report negative emotions around sex and more likely to avoid sexual activity due to embarrassment.[21] The damage to the levator ani plays a critical role in the development of POP, but also this muscle contributes to the orgasmic experience by performing rhythmic muscle contractions.[22] Treatment options should consider the patient's sexual preference because types of pessaries used for the treatment may prohibit penetrative sexual activity and surgery has the risk of disrupting the blood flow to the pelvic tissue, which can decrease genital sensation or cause pain syndromes secondary to adhesions.[22] Although, it is uncertain if that treatment alone restores sexual function.[23]

Treatment

There are generally 4 treatment courses you may discuss with your patient:

1. Expectant management
2. Pelvic floor physical therapy
3. Pessaries
4. Surgery

Expectant Management

Treatment should largely be driven by symptoms and how distressing these are to the patient. If she is not experiencing hydroureteronephrosis, recurrent urinary tract infections, or vaginal or cervical erosions, or infections secondary to the prolapse, expectant management is reasonable.[16] The patient can be counseled on lifestyle modifications, which may include weight loss. Strikingly, a 5% reduction in weight loss can lead to a 50% reduction in pelvic floor dysfunction including urinary incontinence, but the same results have not been shown in improving POP symptoms or reversing herniation.[24] However, one could propose that it could stop the progression and worsening of POP. Also to consider is that prolapse symptoms may worsen with exercise or standing for prolonged periods.

Pelvic Floor Muscle Training

PFMT can be performed either by the medical provider or by a pelvic floor physical therapist. It has been shown to increase pelvic floor muscle strength and endurance as well as decrease the levator hiatus area.[25] In a primary care setting, up to 57% of women reported improvement of symptoms compared with 13% that were in the expectant management group.[17] Furthermore, PFMT improves the prolapse stage by 17% compared with no treatment.[26] When prescribed a regimen by the medical provider, improvements are seen when the patient does 45 to 50 exercises per day divided into 2 or 3 sets.[16] PFMT may improve muscle strength and therefore reduce symptoms associated with POP, but it does not restore the anatomy.[21] A study looked at whether using PFMT pre-POP surgery would improve outcomes, and it did not seem to have a clear benefit.[25,26]

Pessaries

Every woman who has symptomatic POP should be offered a pessary, particularly those who want a nonsurgical option or for which surgery is contraindicated. Pessaries can essentially be divided into 2 categories: pessaries that provide support and pessaries that fill space (**Table 2**). The most common pessaries for POP are the ring pessary and the Gellhorn pessary.[21] Pessaries can be used all the time or as needed, for example, during exercise.

The patient can be fitted with a pessary in the office. When fitting the pessary, the clinician should ask the patient to walk, sit, and void with the pessary in place to make sure this is comfortable for her as well as it fits correctly and does not fall out.[16] Ninety-two percent of women can be successfully fit with a pessary, and many women are quite pleased with it. After 6 months and 1 year of use, 96% and 50% of women were still satisfied with this treatment modality, respectively.[7,11,21] Patients should be educated about removing and cleaning at home daily to weekly; otherwise, she should return to the office every 3 months for removal and cleaning. It is reasonable to start with the ring pessary and move to Gellhorn if the ring pessary does not provide enough support (**Fig. 3**). Some considerations before pessary use include whether she has a chronic condition that may affect pessary use including arthritis, pulmonary disease, obesity, diabetes, pulmonary disease, connective tissue disorder.[27] In a 2007 study, it was found that both types of pessaries provide subjective symptom relief from POP, but only the Gellhorn provided clinically significant improvements in the PFDI-20 scores.[27]

Table 2
Pessaries

Increasing level of support	Support	Space Filling	Sexual Activity Consideration
	Ring Dish Shaatz		Can be used during sexual activity
	Gehrung	Inflatoball Cube	Can be removed for sexual activity
		Gellhorn Poppy Donut	Cannot be sexually active

Most common of these used for POP are ring pessary and Gellhorn pessary. Pessaries can be divided into supportive pessaries versus space filling pessaries In general, the space-filling pessaries are more supportive than the support pessaries. Pessary use is not a contraindication to sexual intercourse, but there are several pessaries that can neither be removed at the time of intercourse, nor can vaginal penetration occur with them in place (Gellhorn, Poppy, Donut).

Data from Radnia N, Hajhashemi M, Eftekhar T, Deldar M, Mohajeri T, Sohbati S, Ghanbari Z. Patient Satisfaction and Symptoms Improvement in Women Using a Vaginal Pessary for The Treatment of Pelvic Organ Prolapse. J Med Life. 2019 Jul-Sep;12(3):271-275. https://doi.org/10.25122/jml-2019-0042. PMID: 31666830; PMCID: PMC6814872

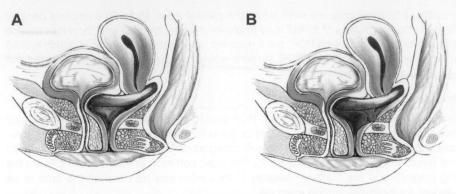

Fig. 3. Ring (*A*) and Gellhorn (*B*) pessaries in a sagittal view. Ring pessary is purely a support pessary, whereas Gellhorn is a space-filling pessary. It is reasonable to try to fit a ring pessary first followed by Gellhorn, as Gellhorn may have more success with severer cases of POP. (Original illustration completed for this manuscript by K. Glen Saldanha, PT, DPT, OCS, TPS.)

Two side effects to counsel patients on are increased vaginal discharge and vaginal erosions. However, vaginal discharge usually improves over time in 6 to 8 months and the use of vaginal estrogen can decrease discharge and erosions.[5,11] Because the pessary needs to be removed and cleaned periodically to prevent infection and erosion of the vaginal canal, a patient who is noncompliant with follow-through is not a good candidate for a pessary. The clinician should also ask about urinary incontinence history. Prolapsed anatomy may obstruct the ureters, which will mask incontinence. When the pessary is inserted (or surgery is performed), urinary incontinence may be unmasked causing bothersome symptoms.[11,27] Another consideration is using pessaries in obese women, who may have relative contraindications to surgery. Even though weight loss may not improve prolapse symptoms or restore normal anatomy, pessaries have been found to be an efficacious treatment modality in obese women.[28]

One may be wondering how pessaries affect sexual activity. Historically, it has been believed that sexual activity is a contraindication to pessary use. Certain pessaries can be used during sexual activity, and others can be removed for sexual activity (**Table 3**). In general, support pessaries can either be removed for vaginal intercourse or maintained in situ for vaginal intercourse, and support pessaries may not be able to be removed and therefore sexual intercourse is contraindicated. The clinician can also counsel patients that pessaries have been shown to improve sexual function, not hinder.[21]

Surgery

Surgery is a common treatment option, especially for higher stages of prolapse or when expectant and conservative management is contraindicated. Women of all ages may seek surgical treatment, a study found that the most common age for surgery was in the menopausal period, and complication rates are highest among elderly aged women.[29] Many surgical options may be considered (see **Table 3**). The first consideration is to understand what anatomy needs to be corrected: does she have an anterior wall, apical, or posterior prolapse, or a combination of these? Second consideration is whether the patient has a uterus or not. If the uterus is present and she has uterine prolapse, a hysterectomy alone is not enough because she will likely suffer apical prolapse posthysterectomy.[7] A procedure such as colpopexy, where the vaginal vault is suspended to the sacrum, or uterosacral ligament suspension is performed to correct the lax ligaments. Furthermore, she may opt to keep her uterus for

Table 3
Types of POP surgeries

Considerations	Procedure	Indication
Uterus sparing procedures	Hysteropexy	Women with apical prolapse who wish to avoid hysterectomy
Uterus sparing,[a] obliterative procedures	Le Fort partial colpoclesis	Obliterative procedure that preserves the uterus but can be used for any type of prolapse. This procedure is irreversible. Lateral canals are left for cervical secretions
	Total colpectomy	Constricted vagina, sutures are used to invert the vagina
Most common procedures	Abdominal sacral colpopexy	For recurrent cystocele, vault or enterocele
	Sacrospinous fixation	Indicated for patients with posthysterectomy vaginal vault prolapse, typically done at the time of hysterectomy
	Anterior vaginal repair/ anterio colporrhaphy	For prolapse of bladder or urethra
	Posterior vaginal repair/ posterior colporrhaphy and perineorrhaphy	Indicated for prolapse of rectum, defects of the perineum, or both
Not routinely recommended anymore due to FDA recall of mesh.	Vaginal repair with synthetic mesh or biologic graft augmentation	Indicated for anterior, apical prolapse

[a] These procedures can also be done posthysterectomy.
Data from Pelvic Organ Prolapse: ACOG Practice Bulletin, Number 214. Obstet Gynecol. 2019 Nov;134(5):e126-e142. https://doi.org/10.1097/AOG.0000000000003519. PMID: 31651832.

fertility preservation, sexuality, or body image considerations, and may undergo hysteropexy. The uterus is believed to have a passive role in prolapse, so a hysterectomy is not necessarily indicated when a patient has uterine prolapse. She should be counseled that hysteropexy compared with hysterectomy plus colpopexy results in shorter operative time, less blood loss, and less surgical cost without differences in prolapse recurrence.[30] A colpoclesis is also uterine sparing, but could also be done for apical prolapse posthysterectomy, and is an obliterative procedure in which the vagina is sutured closed. This could be done partially or completely, but regardless the woman will not be able to have penetrative vaginal intercourse anymore. The partial colpoclesis is done to allow cervical secretions to drain. This operation has the highest cure rate and the lowest morbidity and is particularly a great option for those who are at high risk for more complicated surgical procedures.[7,16]

Before surgery, there should be an evaluation for occult stress urinary incontinence and be sure that all cervical pathologic conditions are up to date. If the patient chooses to undergo uterine-preserving surgery, she should be counseled that she may need a subsequent surgery later in the future for uterine pathologic conditions such as dysfunctional uterine bleeding, endometrial hyperplasia, or endometrial cancer.

There are currently no available transvaginal mesh products for the treatment of POP. In 2008, the food and drug administration (FDA) issued a statement warning about transvaginal mesh for POP stating that serious adverse events were not rare and the use of transvaginal mesh did not have better outcomes than repair without mesh.[31] Furthermore, in 2019, they recalled the remainder of transvaginal mesh products for POP off the market stating that more than 100,000 women had sued manufacturers with complaints of persistent vaginal bleeding or discharge, chronic pelvic pain, or dyspareunia.[32] Those individuals who have mesh in place and are asymptomatic, do not need to do anything differently. It is worth noting that this FDA order does not apply to transvaginal mesh for stress urinary incontinence or transabdominal mesh placement for POP repair.[7]

Prognosis

Consequences of POP include urinary incontinence, voiding dysfunction, complete prolapse of the uterus, which results in ulcerations of the vagina, cervix, or uterus, fecal incontinence, or difficulty with defecation, and sexual dysfunction.[1]

Due to POP likely being due to a problem with the pelvic floor itself, such as a partial or full-thickness tear of pelvic muscle during vaginal delivery or complete denervation, surgery may not correct these deficits. The recurrence rate for prolapse after surgery is 6% to 30%, with reoperation rates as high as 30%.[7,9]

Although the strongest association of prolapse is with the first birth, and the risk of prolapse does increase with subsequent births, it is reasonable to consider pelvic floor physical therapy around the antepartum period. Although we know that PFMT does not necessarily reverse the prolapse stage, it might be able to target the prevention of worsening prolapse and, most importantly, correct some symptoms of prolapse for the patient.

SUMMARY

POP is a common concern among women, the prevalence being 3% to 50% in the general population, depending on how the clinician defines POP. It should be based on symptoms with the examination to support, as women who have prolapse on examination may not have bothersome symptoms and therefore do not need treatment. The POP-Q system should be used to document the level of prolapse, which can be used to assess her response to treatment whether conservative treatment is pursued or surgical treatment is performed. Treatment includes expectant management, PFMT, pessaries, and surgery, with surgery being the first line. Regarding PFMT, there were not any studies at the time of this publication that discussed a specific protocol for POP that can be standardized and used among both primary care providers and physical therapists. All protocols were left up to each physical therapist and based on the case presentation. Although this allows for individualized care, it lends that one must be quite skilled in this area to treat POP. A standardized protocol would help make PFMT available to a variety of clinicians in different practice settings.

It is uncertain if hysterectomy is a risk factor for prolapse, but certainly, if a woman has a uterus, a hysterectomy alone will not correct prolapse. She will need additional procedures at the time of hysterectomy including colpopexy or colporrhaphy. Colpoclesis is an obliterative, irreversible procedure with the highest cure rate and lowest morbidity rate, but she will be unable to have penetrative vaginal intercourse postoperatively. Transvaginal mesh for the repair of POP is no longer available, and as of 2019, the FDA has recalled all of these products. Surgical repair of POP may unmask stress urinary incontinence, so this should be evaluated preoperatively with urodynamics.

Overall, the risk of recurrence is 6% to 30%, which is likely due to the underlying problem being in damage to the levator ani muscle itself. Therefore, surgical correction by suspending the vaginal apex or ligaments may not be enough to continue to offer pelvic support. As the population continues to age, we will see increasing cases of POP. The easiest way to screen for this condition is simply asking if the patient feels a bulge in the vagina. From there, the clinician should believe skilled at offering a variety of treatment options with the ability to counsel the patient on these and place referrals as necessary.

CLINICS CARE POINTS

- Pelvic organ prolapse (POP) is defined by The International Urogynecological Association and International Continence Society as the descent of one or more of the anterior vaginal wall, posterior vaginal wall, the uterus (cervix), or the apex of the vagina (vaginal vault or cuff scar after hysterectomy.
- The pelvic organ prolapse-quantification system should be used as a standard objective way to evaluate the severity of POP but also to track treatment response.
- POP is a clinical diagnosis, without the need for laboratory or imaging in most situations.
- The leading cause of POP is levator ani muscle damage, and increasing parity increases one's risk for developing POP.
- The presenting symptom is a bulging sensation in the vagina.
- Pelvic Floor Distress Inventory-20 and Pelvic Floor Impact Questionnaires-7) are 2 validated questionnaires one may consider using to understand how POP is affecting their quality of life; particularly their body image and sexual function.
- A pessary is a first-line treatment of POP. Most women can be fitted for this in the office. Two side effects to counsel women on are increased vaginal discharge and vaginal erosions. Topical estrogen may help.
- Colpoclesis is an irreversible, obliterative procedure with the highest success rate and lowest morbidity but does not allow patient to have vaginal intercourse thereafter.
- In 2019, the FDA recalled the remainder of transvaginal mesh products for POP repair. This order does not include transvaginal mesh for repair of stress urinary incontinence or transabdominal mesh for POP repair.
- After surgery, the recurrence rate of POP is 6% to 30%.

CLINICS CARE POINTS

- Pelvic organ prolapse is defined by The International Urogynecological Association and International Continence Society as the descent of one or more of the anterior vaginal wall, posterior vaginal wall, the uterus (cervix), or the apex of the vagina (vaginal vault or cuff scar after hysterectomy.

- The POP-Q system should be used as a standard objective way to evaluate the severity of POP but also to track treatment response.

- Pelvic organ prolapse is a clinical diagnosis, without the need for laboratory or imaging in most situations.

- The leading cause of POP is levator ani muscle damage, and increasing parity increases one's risk for developing POP.

- The presenting symptom is a bulging sensation in the vagina.

- Pelvic Floor Distress Inventory (PFDI-20) and Pelvic Floor Impact Questionnaires (PFIQ-7) are 2 validated questionnaires one may consider using to understand how POP is affecting their quality of life; particularly their body image and sexual function.

- A pessary is a first-line treatment of POP. Most women can be fitted for this in the office. Two side effects to counsel women on are increased vaginal discharge and vaginal erosions. Topical estrogen may help.

- Colpoclesis is an irreversible, obliterative procedure with the highest success rate and lowest morbidity but does not allow patient to have vaginal intercourse thereafter.

- In 2019, the FDA recalled the remainder of transvaginal mesh products for POP repair. This order does not include transvaginal mesh for repair of stress urinary incontinence or transabdominal mesh for POP repair.

- After surgery, the recurrence rate of POP is 6% to 30%.

DISCLOSURE

The authors have nothing to disclose.

REFERENCES

1. Hendrix SL, Clark A, Nygaard I, et al. Pelvic organ prolapse in the Women's Health Initiative: gravity and gravidity. Am J Obstet Gynecol 2002;186:1160–6.
2. Vergeldt TF, Weemhoff M, IntHout J, et al. Risk factors for pelvic organ prolapse and its recurrence: a systematic review. Int Urogynecol J 2015;26(11):1559–73.
3. Weintraub AY, Glinter H, Marcus-Braun N. Narrative review of the epidemiology, diagnosis and pathophysiology of pelvic organ prolapse. Int Braz J Urol 2020; 46(1):5–14.
4. DeLancey JO. What's new in the functional anatomy of pelvic organ prolapse? Curr Opin Obstet Gynecol 2016;28(5):420–9.
5. Takacs P, Kozma B, Larson K. Pelvic organ prolapse: from estrogen to pessary. Menopause 2019;26(2):121–2.
6. Haylen BT, de Ridder D, Freeman RM, et al. International Urogynecological Association; International Continence Society. An International Urogynecological Association (IUGA)/International Continence Society (ICS) joint report on the terminology for female pelvic floor dysfunction. Neuroural Urodyn 2010; 29(1):4–20.
7. Pelvic Organ Prolapse: ACOG Practice Bulletin, Number 214. Obstet Gynecol 2019;134(5):e126–42.
8. Madhu C, Swift S, Moloney-Geany S, et al. How to use the Pelvic Organ Prolapse Quantification (POP-Q) system? Neurourol Urodyn 2018;37(S6):S39–43.
9. Ashton-Miller JA, DeLancey JO. Functional anatomy of the female pelvic floor. Ann N Y Acad Sci 2007;1101:266–96.
10. Kieserman-Shmokler C, Swenson CW, Chen L, et al. From molecular to macro: the key role of the apical ligaments in uterovaginal support. Am J Obstet Gynecol 2020;222(5):427–36.
11. Radnia N, Hajhashemi M, Eftekhar T, et al. Patient Satisfaction and Symptoms Improvement in Women Using a Vaginal Pessary for The Treatment of Pelvic Organ Prolapse. J Med Life 2019;12(3):271–5.
12. Delancey JO, Morgan DM, Fenner DE, et al. Comparison of levator ani muscle defects and function in women with and without pelvic organ prolapse. Obstet Gynecol 2007;109(2 pt 1):295–302.

13. Barber MD, Maher C. Epidemiology and outcome assessment of pelvic organ prolapse. Int Urogynecol J 2013;24:1783–90.
14. Nygaard I, Barber MD, Burgio KL, et al. Pelvic Floor Disorders Network. Prevalence of systematic pelvic floor disorders in US women. JAMA 2008;300:1311–6.
15. Wu JM, Vaughn CP, Goode PS, et al. Prevalence and trends of symptomatic pelvic floor disorders in US women. Obstet Gynecol 2014;123(1):141–8.
16. Iglesia CB, Smithling KR. Pelvic Organ Prolapse. Am Fam Physician 2017;96(3): 179–85.
17. Wingers a Man. Panman CM, Kollen BJ. Berger MH. Lisman-Van Leeu-wen Y, Dekker JH. Effect of pelvic floor muscle training compared with watchful waiting in older women with symptomatic mild pelvic organ prolapse: randomized controlled trial in primary care. BMJ 2014;349:g7378.
18. Barber MD, Walters MD, Bump RC. Short forms of two condition-specific quality-of-life questionnaires for women with pelvic floor disorders (PFDI-20 and PFIQ-7). Am J Obstet Gynecol 2005;193(1):103–13.
19. Jelovsek JE, Barber MD. Women seeking treatment for advanced pelvic organ prolapse have decreased body image and quality of life. Am J Obstet Gynecol 2006;194(5):1455–61.
20. Sexual health. World Health Organization. Available at: https://www.who.int/health-topics/sexual-health#tab=tab_2. Accessed July 30, 2021.
21. Rantell A. Vaginal pessaries for pelvic organ prolapse and their impact on sexual function. Sex Med Rev 2019;7(4):597–603.
22. Stein A, Sauder SK, Reale J. The role of physical therapy in sexual health in men and women: evaluation and treatment. Sex Med Rev 2019;7(1):46–56.
23. Handa VL, Cundiff G, Chang HH, et al. Female sexual function and pelvic floor disorders. Obstet Gynecol 2008;111(5):1045–52.
24. Ramalingam K, Monga A. Obesity and pelvic floor dysfunction. Best Pract Res Clin Obstet Gynaecol 2015;29:541–7.
25. Duarte TB, Bø K, Brito LGO, et al. Perioperative pelvic floor muscle training did not improve outcomes in women undergoing pelvic organ prolapse surgery: a randomised trial. J Physiother 2020;66(1):27–32.
26. Hagen S, Stark D. Conservative prevention and management of pelvic organ prolapse in women. Cochrane Database Syst Rev 2011;(12):CD003882.
27. Cundiff GW, Amundsen CL, Bent AE, et al. The PESSRI study: symptom relief outcomes of a randomized crossover trial of the ring and Gellhorn pessaries. Am J Obstet Gynecol 2007;196(4):405.e1-8.
28. de Sam Lazaro S, Nardos R, Caughey AB. Obesity and pelvic floor dysfunction: battling the bulge. Obstet Gynecol Surv 2016;71:114–25.
29. Shah AD, Kohli N, Rajan SS, et al. The age distribution, rates, and types of surgery for pelvic organ prolapse in the USA. Int Urogynecol J Pelvic Floor Dysfunct 2008;19:421–8.
30. Meriwether KV, Antosh DD, Olivera CK, et al. Uterine preservation vs hysterectomy in pelvic organ prolapse surgery: a systematic review with meta-analysis and clinical practice guidelines. Am J Obstet Gynecol 2018;219(2):129–46.e2.
31. Urogynecologic Surgical Mesh: Update on the Safety and Effectiveness of Transvaginal Placement for Pelvic Organ Prolapse. July 2011. Available at: https://www.fda.gov/files/medical%20devices/published/Urogynecologic-Surgical-Mesh%5fUpdate-on-the-Safety-and-Effectiveness-of-Transvaginal-Placement-for-Pelvic-Organ-Prolapse-%28July-2011%29.pdf. Accessed July 30, 2021.
32. Dyer O. Transvaginal mesh: FDA orders remaining products off US market. BMJ 2019;365:l1839.

Pregnancy Loss

Toni Beth Jackson, MMS, PA-C

KEYWORDS

- Early pregnancy loss • Spontaneous abortion • Late pregnancy loss • Miscarriage
- Mid-trimester miscarriage • Second-trimester abortion • Recurrent pregnancy loss
- Stillbirth

KEY POINTS

- Pregnancy loss in the first trimester is more common than at a later stage in pregnancy.
- Early, late, and recurrent pregnancy loss (RPL) have many similar risk factors, although some are specific to each category.
- RPL requires thorough work up for evaluation of comorbid disorders.
- Management of early pregnancy loss can occur in the outpatient setting, whereas late pregnancy loss commonly requires inpatient care.
- Following pregnancy loss, patients are at an increased risk for cardiovascular disease and psychological symptoms.

INTRODUCTION

Loss of a pregnancy at any stage is a common occurrence at a rate of 19.7%, with early pregnancy loss (EPL) being more common than loss at later stages in pregnancy.[1] Pregnancy loss at any stage can be a devastating experience, and there are additional long-term effects, both physical and psychological. Providers must be aware of the risk factors, assessment, and management of pregnancy loss and its sequelae.

DEFINITIONS

The term EPL is defined as loss of a pregnancy in the first trimester, before 12weeks and 6 days gestation.[2,3] EPL occurs at a rate of approximately 13.5%.[1] The term EPL is a hypernym of threatened abortion, incomplete abortion, and complete abortion. A threatened abortion occurs when a patient experiences symptoms of a pregnancy loss, but a viable intrauterine pregnancy (IUP) is still present. However, this is often a precursor to a complete or incomplete abortion.

Incomplete abortion presents with symptoms of pregnancy loss, confirmation of a nonviable IUP, with retention of products of conception in the uterus.[2] This is easily distinguished from a complete abortion, where a patient completely expels the products of conception from the uterus and has a complete resolution of symptoms.

Wake Forest University School of Medicine Department of PA Studies, Medical Center Boulevard, Winston-Salem, NC, 27157, USA
E-mail address: Tbjackso@wakehealth.edu

Physician Assist Clin 7 (2022) 499–511
https://doi.org/10.1016/j.cpha.2022.03.004
2405-7991/22/© 2022 Elsevier Inc. All rights reserved.
physicianassistant.theclinics.com

Late pregnancy loss can be used to broadly describe the loss of an IUP after the first trimester. In most studies on pregnancy loss, the term second trimester miscarriage has been used to describe the death of a fetus after 13 weeks and before 20 weeks gestation, whereas stillbirth is used to describe the death of a fetus after 20 weeks gestation. The term recurrent pregnancy loss (RPL) is used when a patient experiences the loss of two or more pregnancies prior to 20 weeks gestation.[4] A summary of these terms can be found in **Table 1**. Inconsistent terminology exists with regard to pregnancy loss leading to confusion among the public, patients, and providers. Using terminology to categorize the loss based on gestational age and avoiding use of scientific jargon is best practice.

BACKGROUND
Risk Factors of Pregnancy Loss

Early, late, and RPL share many of the same risk factors. Diagnoses of obesity, type 1 or type 2 diabetes, polycystic ovarian syndrome (PCOS), previous gestational diabetes, or impaired glucose tolerance are all associated with an increased risk for pregnancy loss.[5,6] Thyroid gland dysfunction and systemic lupus erythematosus (SLE) are also risk factors for pregnancy loss.[7,8] The exact mechanisms of these associations are unknown, but it is hypothesized that the hormonal and metabolic derangements associated with these conditions are likely to lower the quality of the endometrium, leading to difficulties with successful implantation and continuous nourishment of the pregnancy.

Abnormalities of the uterus are also a risk factor common to pregnancy loss. The uterine congenital anomalies including bicornuate, unicornuate, septate, and arcuate uteri have all been implicated in pregnancy loss.[4,9] Other uterine abnormalities with an association to loss include intrauterine adhesions (Asherman Syndrome) and endometrial polyps. Uterine fibroids (leiomyomas) are implicated as a risk factor for pregnancy loss, although this is debated.[10,11] Diagnosis of subchorionic hematoma at or before 7 weeks gestation is associated with a high correlation with EPL; however, persistence of a hematoma into the second trimester is not associated with late pregnancy loss.[12,13] Conception in a patient with an intrauterine device (IUD) in situ is associated with an increased risk of pregnancy loss and preterm labor or rupture of membranes; however, these risks are significantly decreased with IUD removal early in the pregnancy.[14] The aforementioned abnormalities of the uterus increase the risk of pregnancy loss due to the unfavorable conditions of the endometrium, necessary for the implantation, growth, and development of a pregnancy.

Maternal history of thrombophilias is associated with an increased risk of pregnancy loss. Antiphospholipid antibody syndrome (APS) is the thrombophilia with the strongest association of pregnancy loss in any trimester and RPL.[6,15] The diagnosis of

Table 1	
Terms related to pregnancy loss[1-4]	
Term	**Definition**
Threatened abortion	Symptoms of EPL with viable IUP on ultrasound
Incomplete abortion	Nonviable IUP with POC retained in uterus
Complete abortion	Complete expulsion of POC; symptom resolution
Second trimester miscarriage	Death of a fetus after 13 wk and before 20 wk gestation
Stillbirth	Death of a fetus after 20 wk gestation
RPL	Loss of 2 or more pregnancies before 20 wk gestation

APS is confirmed when anticardiolipin antibodies, lupus anticoagulant, or anti-β2 glycoprotein-1 antibodies are positive. In recurrent and late pregnancy loss, deficiencies in protein C and S are associated with an increased risk, but this is not an association seen in EPL.[6,15] Factor V Leiden, prothrombin G20210A mutation, and antithrombin deficiency are all risk factors for pregnancy loss but are particularly associated with an increase in late pregnancy loss.[15] Another inherited thrombophilia, methylene tetrahydrofolate reductase (MTHFR) enzyme homozygosity, has been weakly associated with early, late, and RPL, but current evidence is conflicting.[15] The hypothesized cause of pregnancy loss associated with thrombophilia is the increased risk of clot formation within placental vasculature leading to placental insufficiency, intrauterine growth restriction, and preeclampsia.

Certain factors of previous obstetric history can affect pregnancy outcomes. A history of previous pregnancy loss in any trimester is a risk factor for a recurrence, and this risk increases with each subsequent pregnancy loss.[16] Previous caesarean section and preterm delivery are also associated risk factors for subsequent pregnancy loss.[16]

Maternal age at conception has an impact on pregnancy outcome. The lowest risk of pregnancy loss is maternal age between 25 and 29 years, with an increase in the risk of pregnancy loss in women aged 19 years and younger, and in women older than 30 years.[16] As maternal age increases more than 30 years, the risk of pregnancy loss incrementally increases. The highest risk of pregnancy loss being more than 50% in women aged 45 years and older.[16] Paternal age can also be a risk factor, independent of the maternal age. It has been shown that an increased paternal age of 40 years or older is associated with an increased risk of early or late pregnancy loss.[17] Paternal factors are currently being studied with regard to RPL.

Race and ethnicity also are associated with an increased risk of pregnancy loss. In the United States, for example, rates of pregnancy loss were higher among non-Hispanic black and white women when compared with Hispanic women, however, black women have an increased incidence when compared with white women.[1,18] The underlying mechanisms behind these disparities are unclear.

There are several modifiable risk factors that are associated with an increased risk of pregnancy loss. Maternal BMI, both in underweight and overweight categories, specifically BMI ≥25 or less than 18.5 is associated with an increased risk.[19] Elevated BMI (≥25) is a consistent risk factor for patients with RPL.[6] Alcohol use during pregnancy is one of the highest modifiable risk factors of pregnancy loss. Abstaining from alcohol use during pregnancy has been shown to reduce the risk of pregnancy loss by approximately 9%.[19] Substance use in pregnancy including tobacco, cocaine, methamphetamine, and cannabis has been linked to an increased risk of loss.[20,21] Patients must be educated of these modifiable risk factors to reduce the risk adverse pregnancy outcomes.

The use of specific medications during pregnancy has been associated with pregnancy loss. The use of nonsteroidal anti-inflammatory drugs near the time of conception has been associated with EPL.[22] The antibiotic classes of macrolides, sulfonamides, tetracyclines, fluoroquinolones, and metronidazole have also been associated with an increase in pregnancy loss.[23] Prepregnancy counseling and judicious use of antibiotics can avoid this risk.

Social factors can affect the risk of pregnancy loss. Maternal stress has been studied as a risk factor for pregnancy loss. Evidence of this is conflicting, but women experiencing life adversities in the substance abuse or legal domains could be at increased risk for pregnancy loss.[24] Recently, the association of adverse childhood experiences (ACEs) and pregnancy loss have been researched and women with a history of physical and emotional abuse as a child had an increased risk of early and late pregnancy loss.[25] This has not been studied in patients with RPL. Further research is needed to explore the pathophysiological mechanisms associated with this increased risk in patients with stress and history of adversity. A summary of risk factors associated with pregnancy loss is outlined in **Table 2**. Risk factors specific to early, late, or RPL only are discussed in the subsequent section.

Table 2
Risk factors associated with pregnancy loss[4–25,43]

	Risk Factor for Early, Late, and RPL	Early Pregnancy Loss Only	Late Pregnancy Loss Only	RPL Only
Endocrine Disorders	Type 1 and 2 diabetes Impaired glucose tolerance Thyroid disease PCOS Gestational diabetes			
Uterine Abnormalities	Uterine adhesions Endometrial polyps [a]Uterine fibroids Congenital uterine anomalies IUD in situ	Subchorionic hematoma	Cervical insufficiency FGR Umbilical cord anomalies	Cervical insufficiency FGR
Thrombophilias	APS Factor V Leiden Antithrombin deficiency Prothrombin G20210 A mutation [a]MTHFR homozygosity		Protein C and S deficiency	
Other Comorbid Conditions	SLE		Hypertensive disorders Multiple gestation FGR Renal disease Pregnancy achieved with in vitro fertilization	
Past Obstetric History	Prior pregnancy loss Stillbirth Preterm delivery Caesarean section			
Nonmodifiable Risk factors	Age <20 y Age >30 y Black Race	Paternal age ≥40 ACEs		
Modifiable risk factors	Alcohol, tobacco, cocaine, methamphetamine, marijuana use in pregnancy BMI ≥25 or <18.5 [a]Stress Some antibiotic classes	NSAID use in first trimester		

[a] Conflicting data exists regarding impact on pregnancy loss.

DISCUSSION
Pathophysiology of Early Pregnancy Loss

The cause of EPL has been attributed to multiple underlying mechanisms. The most common underlying cause of EPL is chromosomal abnormalities with 70% to 82% of EPL cases having an abnormal karyotype.[26,27] Of these, nearly 65% are due to a single autosomal trisomy such as trisomy 15, 16, 21, or 22.[26] EPL due to a chromosomal abnormality typically occurs earlier in the pregnancy, before 9 weeks gestation. There is a higher correlation of chromosomal abnormality being a leading cause of EPL in mothers of older maternal age.

Immunologic causes of EPL are associated with the inability to halt the mechanisms of the immune system designed to fight against foreign invaders, a paradoxic need for a successful pregnancy. In a healthy pregnancy, a mother's immune system is prevented from attacking the embryo, carrying nonself genetic information. When these complex immunologic mechanisms are not silenced, there is an association with pregnancy loss.[28] Another immunologic cause of pregnancy loss is related to the decidualization, or remodeling, of the endometrium, a process balanced by hormonal and uterine immunologic factors.[29] An imbalance of this process leads to the development of an endometrium that is unfavorable and more likely to result in an EPL.

Another common cause of pregnancy loss is the presence of an infection. If infection is transmitted to the utero-placental unit, the immune responses that occur can disrupt implantation, the formation of or overall health of the placenta. If infection is severe enough to cause sepsis, the subsequent hemodynamic collapse can lead to pregnancy loss. Viruses associated with pregnancy loss include cytomegalovirus (CMV), rubella, dengue fever, and human immunodeficiency virus.[30,31] Other viruses such as human papillomavirus, herpes simplex virus 1 and 2, parvovirus B19, hepatitis B, and polyomavirus BK have been implicated, but evidence of their association is conflicting. Bacterial causes of pregnancy loss include Brucella, Treponema pallidum, Ureaplasma urealyticum, and Mycoplasma hominis. Chlamydia trachomatis has also been implicated, but evidence of its association is conflicting.[31] Malaria, is clearly associated with pregnancy loss while toxoplasmosis, another commonly associated protozoan infection, has conflicting evidence of its association with EPL.[31] Screening and subsequent treatment of these infections in high-risk individuals during pregnancy can reduce the risk of these infections leading to an adverse pregnancy outcome.

Presentation of Early Pregnancy Loss

Vaginal bleeding associated with pelvic pain is a common presentation of EPL. Pelvic pain by itself is not associated with EPL.[32] Vomiting in the first trimester of pregnancy is a symptom with an inverse relationship with pregnancy loss, and its presence is reassuring.[32] Nearly 38% patients may be asymptomatic, and pregnancy loss is identified incidentally on ultrasound.[33] This has been referred to as a "missed-abortion," but is more accurately described as an asymptomatic incomplete abortion.

In a patient with a possible EPL, the hemodynamic status of the patient should be evaluated, ensuring stability before the performance of additional physical examination. In a stable patient, a speculum examination is warranted. Bleeding or tissue in the vagina is a common finding, and the cervical os is most commonly dilated, but a closed cervical os does not rule out a pregnancy loss.

Bimanual examination is also indicated in a patient with suspected pregnancy loss, which can help evaluate for cervical dilation, as well as adnexal or cervical motion tenderness, commonly seen in patients with ectopic pregnancy. Fundal height measurement may be helpful to correlate with gestational age. Fetal heart tones assessment by Doppler can be attempted and if present, would decrease the likelihood of EPL.

Diagnostic Evaluation for Early Pregnancy Loss

The initial diagnostic evaluation in a patient with possible EPL includes obtaining a quantitative beta- human chorionic gonadotropin (β-HCG), complete blood count, and confirmation of Rh status. If signs or symptoms of hemodynamic instability is present, a blood type and cross as well as diagnostics evaluating for disseminated intravascular coagulopathy including prothrombin time (PT), partial thromboplastin time (PTT), fibrinogen, and d-dimer should be performed. Because of the similar presentation, other diagnoses such as ectopic pregnancy and hydatidiform mole (molar pregnancy) must be ruled out in patients presenting with a possible pregnancy loss. This is easily done by using transvaginal ultrasonography. Viability of the embryo must also be evaluated by first inspecting for a fetal heartbeat. If no fetal heartbeat is present, but there is a fetal pole, measure the crown-rump length (CRL). If CRL is ≥ 7 mm with no cardiac activity, this is highly suspicious of EPL.[3] If a gestational sac is present, measuring ≥25 mm but has no fetal pole, this is also highly suggestive of EPL.[3] If abnormal findings are seen, a repeat ultrasound in 7 to 10 days or a repeat quantitative β-HCG in 48 to 72 hours will confirm the diagnosis. Doubling of the quantitative β-HCG level in 48 hours is reassuring of viability.[34] The use of serum progesterone levels alone is not recommended in the diagnosis of EPL, however if less than 35 nmol/L is highly associated with EPL.[35]

Management of Early Pregnancy Loss

Expectant management is the preferred choice for management of EPL and can be used in a patient who is clinically stable, provided that the patient is educated on the expected progression, close follow-up parameters, and pain control management. An Rh-negative patient experiencing EPL who has a negative antibody screen should receive Rho(d) immune globulin within 72 hours to reduce the risk of alloimmunization.[2] An Rh-positive patient who experiences a complete abortion will need no further medical or surgical intervention. If after 7 to 14 days of expectant management the patient is still symptomatic, or if the patient never experienced symptoms, the patient should receive a repeat ultrasonography because this would suggest an incomplete abortion.[3] Medical management options should be discussed with a patient with an incomplete abortion. Single-dose mifepristone 200 mg orally taken 7 to 20 hours before a single dose of misoprostol 800 mcg vaginally can be used to aid in the expulsion of retained products of conception and can be done in an outpatient setting.[2] Vaginal misoprostol can be used alone if mifepristone is unavailable and can be repeated within 1 week if the products of conception are still retained and the patient is afebrile.[2] Surgical intervention with dilation and curettage is required in patients with significant hemorrhaging, hemodynamic compromise, or if signs of sepsis are present.[2] Cervical dilation and suction curettage with or without sharp curettage is the preferred surgical management.[2] To ensure complete resolution of EPL, follow-up ultrasonography or serial quantitative β-HCG is recommended.

Recurrent Pregnancy Loss

RPL, defined as having 2 or more losses, has an estimated incidence of 2.6%.[36] Although patients with recurrent loss share many of the same risk factors with those experiencing early or late pregnancy loss, there are some risk factors that are more specific to RPL. Thirty-eight percentage of patients with a history of RPL have an endocrine disorder, with PCOS being the most common.[6] Structural uterine factors most prevalent in RPL include cervical insufficiency, but other anomalies of the uterus previously mentioned in **Table 2** are also common and considered a risk factor. Thrombophilia risk factors specific to RPL include APS and protein C and S deficiencies, the latter of which is specific to late pregnancy loss and RPL.[6]

Diagnostic Evaluation of Recurrent Pregnancy Loss

Following 2 consecutive pregnancy losses at any stage, a formal workup for RPL is indicated. This includes a thorough history and physical examination exploring possible uterine or endocrine disorders. Early diagnostic evaluation in a patient with RPL includes maternal testing for thyroid stimulating hormone, diabetes screening, prolactin, antiphospholipid antibodies such as anticardiolipin, Lupus anticoagulant, and anti-β_2 glycoprotein-I antibodies.[37] In patients with known family history of thrombophilia or personal history of thromboembolism, evaluation for thrombophilias including factor V Leiden, prothrombin gene mutations, protein C, S, and antithrombin deficiencies are recommended. There is a debate on the role of screening for MTHFR mutations, and it is not currently recommended.[38] Maternal evaluation of uterine abnormalities is also recommended in a patient with RPL, using sonohysterography or hysterosalpingography. The diagnostic workup also includes parental karyotyping to detect chromosomal abnormalities as well as chromosomal analysis of products of conception. The chromosomal analysis of POC have a similar percentage of chromosomal abnormality as those found in EPL in general, again, with single autosomal trisomy being the most common.[39] It is important to note that nearly half of all RPLs will have an unknown cause, despite a thorough workup.

Management of Recurrent Pregnancy Loss

Treatment of RPL depends on the underlying cause, if identified. If parental karyotyping or chromosomal analysis of products of conception are found to be abnormal, genetic counseling referral is initiated. Egg or sperm donation or surrogacy can be options to patients with these underlying genetic predispositions. If underlying endocrine disorder is identified such as thyroid disease or diabetes, strict management of these conditions is recommended to enhance the success of pregnancy. In patients with uterine abnormalities, surgical management can be offered, but the risk reduction of RPL this brings is debated.[37] APS can be treated with daily low-dose aspirin and twice daily unfractionated heparin, and this combination has improved pregnancy outcomes in these patients.[37] Lifestyle modifications including maintaining a healthy weight, abstaining from tobacco, alcohol, and drug use, and maintaining good control over preexisting medical conditions including hypertension, diabetes, and other endocrine disorders are imperative in the management of patients with RPL.

Late Pregnancy Loss

Late pregnancy loss, including second trimester miscarriage and stillbirth, are far less frequent than EPL with an incidence of approximately 5% to 6%.[1,40] The most

Table 3 Infections associated with late pregnancy loss[42,43]	
Bacterial	**Viral**
Group B Streptococcus	CMV
Escherichia coli	Parvovirus B19
Enterococcus	Zika
Listeria monocytogenes	Rift Valley fever virus
T. pallidum	

common causes associated with late pregnancy loss are cervical insufficiency, infection, trauma, genetic abnormalities, and placental anomalies. Cervical insufficiency, the leading cause of second trimester miscarriage, can lead to premature delivery of a fetus before viability.[40] The pathophysiology behind cervical insufficiency is unclear, but associated risk factors include history of cervical conization, loop electrosurgical excision procedure (LEEP), or cervical lacerations.[41] Various bacterial and viral infections are associated with an increased risk of loss in the second trimester and are summarized in **Table 3**.[42] Infection can cause maternal sepsis and hemodynamic instability or infection of the placenta and/or fetus, leading to placental insufficiency or preterm birth.

Trauma to the abdomen is another cause of late pregnancy loss, and the possibility of intimate partner violence must be explored. Chromosomal and genetic abnormalities such as anencephaly, renal agenesis, Turner syndrome, single autosomal trisomies, hydrops fetalis, lethal skeletal dysplasias, are some of the fetal malformations associated with late pregnancy loss.[44]

A healthy placenta allowing the fetus to be provided with sufficient nutrients and oxygen for growth is necessary for a healthy pregnancy. Placental insufficiency describes the conditions where the placenta is too small or is not functioning well enough to support the growth of the growing fetus with appropriate nutrients and blood flow. This leads to fetal growth restriction (FGR), the most common risk factor for stillbirth. Impairment of the placenta may be a contributing factor in late pregnancy loss even when other causes are identified.[45] Placental anomalies common in second trimester miscarriage include placenta previa, subchorionic hematomas, and subchorionic thromboses, all of which can cause some degree of placental insufficiency.[43] Other maternal conditions that can lead to placental insufficiency or FGR include chronic hypertension, gestational hypertension, preeclampsia, diabetes mellitus, SLE, renal disease, substance use, preeclampsia, and thrombophilias.[46] Placental abruption is another common cause of stillbirth, and is attributed to maternal cocaine or tobacco use.

Presentation and Evaluation of Late Pregnancy Loss

Many of the common causes of late pregnancy loss have risk factors that can be evaluated before loss. For example, FGR can be identified with fundal height measurement and ultrasonography and monitored throughout the pregnancy. Similarly, cervical insufficiency, the most common cause of second trimester miscarriage, presents with cervical dilation without contractions. Some patients may present with signs of preterm labor including uterine contractions with cervical effacement or dilation of at least 2 cm.[47] Patients may also present with preterm premature rupture of membranes (PPROM). This presentation is more common in patients with underlying infectious cause such as chorioamnionitis, and these patients may also have symptoms of fever, pelvic pain, or uterine contractions as a result of the infection. Some patients with PPROM have no cause identified. Similar to EPL, some patients present with pelvic pain and vaginal bleeding. A history of diminished sensation of fetal movements or inability to find fetal heart tones during routine obstetric appointment may be the only indications of a late pregnancy loss.

Initial diagnostic evaluation of a patient with late pregnancy loss is the confirmation of fetal death via ultrasonography, followed by routine laboratory work including complete blood count, confirmation of Rh status, and blood type and cross if hemodynamic instability is present. An Rh-negative patient should receive Rho(d) immune globulin to reduce the risk of alloimmunization. Amniocentesis before delivery for fetal karyotype testing can be offered. Maternal screening tests for fetal–maternal hemorrhage, syphilis, and antiphospholipid antibodies should also be performed at the time of demise.[43] If placental abruption is identified, toxicology screen is indicated.

Management of Late Pregnancy Loss

Management of late pregnancy loss depends on factors of patient presentation. Patients with cervical insufficiency can be monitored with ultrasonography to assess the need for management. Cervical cerclage can be performed in women prophylactically at 13 to 14 weeks gestation if they have a history of 1 or more second trimester pregnancy losses related to painless cervical dilation.[41] Similarly, if a patient presents in the second trimester with a history and physical examination of painless cervical dilation in the absence of contractions, cervical cerclage can be placed; however, outcomes are varied.[41]

Preterm labor occurring before fetal viability presents ethically complex challenges. For example, patients presenting with preterm labor before 34 weeks gestation are technically not candidates for tocolytic therapy because the risk of fetal morbidity and mortality is high with or without tocolysis.[47] However, each patient must be counseled on risks and benefits to both mother and fetus of interventions that are available. Such treatment options include short-term tocolytic therapy to allow for corticosteroid administration needed for premature lungs and magnesium sulfate needed for neurologic protection, and antibiotic treatment in the event of PPROM.[48] If intervention is agreed on, it is important that the infrastructure needed to deliver the most optimal maternal and neonatal care is available. Similarly, parents must be educated of the likelihood of survival and the risk of chronic disability, which largely depends on the gestational age of delivery. One tool that can be used to predict the outcome of periviable delivery is the Extremely Preterm Birth Outcomes Tool, which calculates the average survival and developmental outcomes at 18 to 26 months of age based on gestational age.[49]

In a patient with fetal death confirmed with ultrasonography, delivery of the fetus and products of conception must be performed and is typically done in an inpatient setting. Before 20 weeks gestation, mifepristone with misoprostol management can be used as a method for induction, similar to the management of EPL.[43] Between 20 and 28 weeks gestation, vaginal misoprostol alone or oxytocin infusion can be used for labor induction, and after 28 weeks gestation oxytocin infusion is used for induction.[43] Although induction and delivery allows the parents with the opportunity to hold their infant, when pregnancy loss occurs before 24 weeks, this procedure is associated with an increased risk for maternal infection requiring antibiotic treatment and patients may also require a follow-up dilation and curettage for removal of placenta after delivery of the fetus.[43] Dilation and evacuation can also be offered; however, this can limit the ability to perform a thorough fetal analysis and autopsy and does not always provide parents the opportunity to hold the infant.[43] Following delivery, fetal autopsy and placental examination by a pathologist can be performed and will often times provide valuable information that can help with identifying the underlying cause.

Recurrent Late Pregnancy Loss

Previous history of pregnancy loss is a risk factor for subsequent pregnancy loss. In the setting of late pregnancy loss, the incidence of recurrence is approximately 4%.[44] Although previous late pregnancy loss increases the risk of recurrent late pregnancy loss, it is not associated with an increased risk of EPL.[44] Recurrent late pregnancy loss is more likely due to maternal or placental causes, such as infection, preterm labor, PPROM, placental insufficiency, or abruption, rather than fetal abnormalities.[44] Diagnostic evaluation of recurrent late pregnancy loss is the same as in recurrent EPL, with the addition of pathologic condition evaluation of fetus and placenta, if available.

Sequelae of Pregnancy Loss

The loss of a pregnancy at any stage can be devastating and traumatic. Providers must also support patients and their families following the traumatic loss with options to assist with their bereavement that best fit their needs. These options include pregnancy loss support groups, bereavement counseling, and referral to other mental health professionals if necessary. Symptoms of anxiety, posttraumatic stress disorder, and depression are common following pregnancy loss and the risk of suicide is increased.[36] The risk of developing major depression following pregnancy loss is twice as high in black women than nonblack women.[50] It is imperative that all patients with pregnancy loss be evaluated for the mental health disorders that may present in the months following the loss and treated appropriately.

In patients with a history of pregnancy loss, there is also increased risk of many other health conditions. In subsequent pregnancies, the risk is increased for RPL, still birth, or preterm labor. This risk for preterm labor following pregnancy loss is strongest in black women.[18] Long-term health problems that are associated with pregnancy loss include increased cardiovascular risk. For example, there is an increased incidence of hypertension, ischemic heart disease, hypercholesterolemia, as well as type II diabetes in patients with a history of pregnancy loss.[51,52]

SUMMARY

Providers must be prepared to educate and manage patients with pregnancy loss at any stage of pregnancy. This outcome of pregnancy, although common, must be approached with empathy and clear communication of risks, benefits, and options in their evaluation and management so that shared decision-making can best take place.

CLINICS CARE POINTS

- Patient education on modifiable risk factors of pregnancy loss including obesity, use of certain medications, tobacco, alcohol, cannabis, cocaine, and methamphetamine should be given at preconception and prenatal visits.

- When evaluating a patient with a possible early pregnancy loss (EPL), assess for signs of hemodynamic instability, obtain a quantitative β-HCG, Rh factor, and perform a transvaginal ultrasonography.

- In a stable patient with an EPL, expectant management is the treatment of choice; however, medical management with oral mifepristone followed by intravaginal misoprostol can be used in the setting of incomplete abortion.

- After 2 pregnancy losses, an evaluation for underlying uterine, endocrine, hematologic, and genetic disorders should be performed.

- Following pregnancy loss at any stage, Rh-negative patients should receive Rho(d) immune globulin.

- Management of late pregnancy loss requires expulsion of the fetus and products of conception, but the method depends on the gestational age of the fetus.

- A patient with a history of pregnancy loss is at an increased risk for mental health conditions, a subsequent pregnancy loss, and cardiovascular disease.

DISCLOSURE

The author has nothing to disclose.

REFERENCES

1. Rossen LM, Ahrens KA, Branum AM. Trends in Risk of Pregnancy Loss Among US Women, 1990–2011. Paediatr Perinat Epidemiol 2018;32(1):19–29.
2. ACOG Practice Bulletin No. 200 Summary: Early Pregnancy Loss. Obstet Gynecol 2018;132(5):1311–3.
3. Overview | Ectopic pregnancy and miscarriage: diagnosis and initial management | Guidance | NICE. Available at: https://www.nice.org.uk/guidance/ng126. Accessed July 20, 2021.
4. The ESHRE Guideline Group on RPL, Bender Atik R, Christiansen OB, et al. ESHRE guideline: recurrent pregnancy loss. Hum Reprod Open 2018;2018(2). https://doi.org/10.1093/hropen/hoy004.
5. Ornoy A, Becker M, Weinstein-Fudim L, et al. Diabetes during Pregnancy: A Maternal Disease Complicating the Course of Pregnancy with Long-Term Deleterious Effects on the Offspring. A Clinical Review. Int J Mol Sci 2021;22(6):2965.
6. Matjila MJ, Hoffman A, van der Spuy ZM. Medical conditions associated with recurrent miscarriage—Is BMI the tip of the iceberg? Eur J Obstet Gynecol Reprod Biol 2017;214:91–6.
7. Dhillon-Smith RK, Tobias A, Smith PP, et al. The Prevalence of Thyroid Dysfunction and Autoimmunity in Women With History of Miscarriage or Subfertility. J Clin Endocrinol Metab 2020;105(8):2667–77.
8. D'Ippolito S, Ticconi C, Tersigni C, et al. The pathogenic role of autoantibodies in recurrent pregnancy loss. Am J Reprod Immunol 2020;83(1):e13200.
9. Chan YY, Jayaprakasan K, Tan A, et al. Reproductive outcomes in women with congenital uterine anomalies: a systematic review. Ultrasound Obstet Gynecol 2011;38(4):371–82.
10. Young BK. A multidisciplinary approach to pregnancy loss: the pregnancy loss prevention center. J Perinat Med 2019;47(1):41–4.
11. Sundermann AC, Velez Edwards DR, Bray MJ, et al. Leiomyomas in Pregnancy and Spontaneous Abortion: A Systematic Review and Meta-analysis. Obstet Gynecol 2017;130(5):1065–72.
12. Heller HT, Asch EA, Durfee SM, et al. Subchorionic Hematoma: Correlation of Grading Techniques With First-Trimester Pregnancy Outcome. J Ultrasound Med 2018;37(7):1725–32.
13. Naert MN, Khadraoui H, Muniz Rodriguez A, et al. Association Between First-Trimester Subchorionic Hematomas and Pregnancy Loss in Singleton Pregnancies. Obstet Gynecol 2019;134(2):276–81.
14. Brahmi D, Steenland MW, Renner R-M, et al. Pregnancy outcomes with an IUD in situ: a systematic review. Contraception 2012;85(2):131–9.
15. Simcox LE, Ormesher L, Tower C, et al. Thrombophilia and Pregnancy Complications. Int J Mol Sci 2015;16(12):28418–28.
16. Magnus MC, Wilcox AJ, Morken N-H, et al. Role of maternal age and pregnancy history in risk of miscarriage: prospective register based study. BMJ 2019;364: l869.
17. du Fossé NA, van der Hoorn M-LP, van Lith JMM, et al. Advanced paternal age is associated with an increased risk of spontaneous miscarriage: a systematic review and meta-analysis. Hum Reprod Update 2020;26(5):650–69.

18. Oliver-Williams CT, Steer PJ. Racial variation in the number of spontaneous abortions before a first successful pregnancy, and effects on subsequent pregnancies. Int J Gynecol Obstet 2015;129(3):207–12.

19. Nilsson SF, Andersen PK, Strandberg-Larsen K, et al. Risk factors for miscarriage from a prevention perspective: a nationwide follow-up study. BJOG Int J Obstet Gynaecol 2014;121(11):1375–85.

20. Coleman-Cowger VH, Oga E, Peters EN, et al. Prevalence and Associated Birth Outcomes of Co-Use of Cannabis and Tobacco Cigarettes during Pregnancy. Neurotoxicol Teratol 2018;68:84–90.

21. Ness RB, Grisso JA, Hirschinger N, et al. Cocaine and Tobacco Use and the Risk of Spontaneous Abortion. Available at: https://doi.org/10.1056/NEJM199902043400501. doi:10.1056/NEJM199902043400501

22. Li D-K, Ferber JR, Odouli R, et al. Use of nonsteroidal antiinflammatory drugs during pregnancy and the risk of miscarriage. Am J Obstet Gynecol 2018;219(3):275.e1-8.

23. Muanda FT, Sheehy O, Bérard A. Use of antibiotics during pregnancy and risk of spontaneous abortion. CMAJ Can Med Assoc J 2017;189(17):E625–33.

24. Li Y, Margerison-Zilko C, Strutz KL, et al. Life Course Adversity and Prior Miscarriage in a Pregnancy Cohort. Womens Health Issues 2018;28(3):232–8.

25. Kerkar S, Shankar A, Boynton-Jarrett R, et al. Adverse Childhood Experiences are Associated with Miscarriage in Adulthood: The GROWH Study. Matern Child Health J 2021;25(3):479–86.

26. Soler A, Morales C, Mademont-Soler I, et al. Overview of Chromosome Abnormalities in First Trimester Miscarriages: A Series of 1,011 Consecutive Chorionic Villi Sample Karyotypes. Cytogenet Genome Res 2017;152(2):81–9.

27. Ozawa N, Ogawa K, Sasaki A, et al. Maternal age, history of miscarriage, and embryonic/fetal size are associated with cytogenetic results of spontaneous early miscarriages. J Assist Reprod Genet 2019;36(4):749–57.

28. Deshmukh H, Way SS. Immunological basis for recurrent fetal loss and pregnancy complications. Annu Rev Pathol 2019;14:185–210.

29. The Annual Capri Workshop Group. Early pregnancy loss: the default outcome for fertilized human oocytes. J Assist Reprod Genet 2020;37(5):1057–63.

30. Oliveira GM de, Pascoal-Xavier MA, Moreira DR, et al. Detection of cytomegalovirus, herpes virus simplex, and parvovirus b19 in spontaneous abortion placentas. J Matern Fetal Neonatal Med 2019;32(5):768–75.

31. Giakoumelou S, Wheelhouse N, Cuschieri K, et al. The role of infection in miscarriage. Hum Reprod Update 2016;22(1):116–33.

32. Sapra KJ, Buck Louis GM, Sundaram R, et al. Signs and symptoms associated with early pregnancy loss: findings from a population-based preconception cohort. Hum Reprod Oxf Engl 2016;31(4):887–96.

33. Linnakaari R, Helle N, Mentula M, et al. Trends in the incidence, rate and treatment of miscarriage—nationwide register-study in Finland, 1998–2016. Hum Reprod 2019. https://doi.org/10.1093/humrep/dez211. dez211.

34. Puget C, Joueidi Y, Bauville E, et al. Serial hCG and progesterone levels to predict early pregnancy outcomes in pregnancies of uncertain viability: A prospective study. Eur J Obstet Gynecol Reprod Biol 2018;220:100–5.

35. Lek SM, Ku CW, Allen JC Jr, et al. Validation of serum progesterone <35nmol/L as a predictor of miscarriage among women with threatened miscarriage. BMC Pregnancy Childbirth 2017;17(1):78.

36. Quenby S, Gallos ID, Dhillon-Smith RK, et al. Miscarriage matters: the epidemiological, physical, psychological, and economic costs of early pregnancy loss. Lancet 2021;397(10285):1658–67.
37. Shahine L, Lathi R. Recurrent Pregnancy Loss: Evaluation and Treatment. Obstet Gynecol Clin North Am 2015;42(1):117–34.
38. ACOG Practice Bulletin No. 197: Inherited Thrombophilias in Pregnancy. Obstet Gynecol 2018;132(1):e18.
39. Popescu F, Jaslow CR, Kutteh WH. Recurrent pregnancy loss evaluation combined with 24-chromosome microarray of miscarriage tissue provides a probable or definite cause of pregnancy loss in over 90% of patients. Hum Reprod 2018; 33(4):579–87.
40. Joubert M, Sibiude J, Bounan S, et al. Mid-trimester miscarriage and subsequent pregnancy outcomes: the role of cervical insufficiency in a cohort of 175 cases. J Matern Fetal Neonatal Med 2021;1–6. https://doi.org/10.1080/14767058.2020.1861600.
41. Practice Bulletin No. 142: Cerclage for the Management of Cervical Insufficiency. Obstet Gynecol 2014;123(2 PART 1):372–9.
42. Page JM, Bardsley T, Thorsten V, et al. Stillbirth Associated With Infection in a Diverse U.S. Cohort. Obstet Gynecol 2019;134(6):1187–96.
43. Management of Stillbirth: Obstetric Care Consensus No, 10. Obstet Gynecol 2020;135(3):e110.
44. McPherson E. Recurrence of stillbirth and second trimester pregnancy loss. Am J Med Genet A 2016;170(5):1174–80.
45. McPherson E. Fetoplacental ratios in stillbirths and second trimester miscarriages. Am J Med Genet A 2020;182(2):322–7.
46. ACOG Practice Bulletin No. 204: Fetal Growth Restriction. Obstet Gynecol 2019; 133(2):e97.
47. Practice Bulletin No. 171: Management of Preterm Labor. Obstet Gynecol 2016; 128(4):e155.
48. Obstetric Care Consensus No. 6: Periviable Birth. Obstet Gynecol 2017;130(4): e187.
49. Extremely Preterm Birth Outcomes Tool. Available at: https://www.nichd.nih.gov/ https://www.nichd.nih.gov/research/supported/EPBO. Accessed September 6, 2021.
50. Shorter JM, Koelper N, Sonalkar S, et al. Racial Disparities in Mental Health Outcomes Among Women With Early Pregnancy Loss. Obstet Gynecol 2021;137(1): 156–63.
51. HORN J, TANZ LJ, STUART JJ, et al. Early or Late Pregnancy Loss and Development of Clinical Cardiovascular Disease Risk Factors: a Prospective Cohort Study. BJOG Int J Obstet Gynaecol 2019;126(1):33–42.
52. Wagner MM, Bhattacharya S, Visser J, et al. Association between miscarriage and cardiovascular disease in a Scottish cohort. Heart 2015;101(24):1954–60.

Gestational Trophoblastic Disease and Neoplasia

Kimberly Weikel, MPAS, PA-C[a],*, Elyse Watkins, DHSc, PA-C, DFAAPA, NCMP[b]

KEYWORDS

- Molar pregnancy • Complete mole • Partial mole • Hydatidiform mole
- Gestational trophoblastic disease • Gestational trophoblastic neoplasia
- Aberrant fertilization

KEY POINTS

- Gestational trophoblastic disease can easily be diagnosed during the first trimester with the use of ultrasound imaging.
- Patients with complete moles almost always present with vaginal bleeding between 6 and 16 weeks; thus, this should always be high on the differential diagnosis. Prompt referral to gynecologic oncology is essential as they have a high risk of malignant transformation.
- Partial moles are more likely to present with a small for gestational age uterus and hCG levels rarely exceeding 100,000 mIU/mL. The risk for malignant transformation is much smaller with a partial mole.
- Complete moles are more likely to present with a large for gestational age uterus with multiple theca lutein ovarian cysts. In addition, complete moles will present with hCG levels greater than 100,000 mIU/mL.
- Patients with complete or partial moles must undergo dilation and curettage. Gestational trophoblastic neoplasia can occur as a consequence of partial or complete moles thus requiring close monitoring from gynecologic oncology.

INTRODUCTION

This article provides an overview of gestational trophoblastic disease (GTD) and gestational trophoblastic neoplasia (GTN) so that providers can promptly diagnose and initiate an appropriate work-up in anticipation of managing or referring to gynecologic oncology. The current recommendations regarding patient education and surveillance are also discussed.

[a] Department of Obstetrics and Gynecology, University of Colorado Anschutz Campus, Mail stop B198-2 Academic Office 1 12631 East, 17th Avenue, Room. 4-2111 Aurora, CO 80045, USA;
[b] University of Lynchburg, 1501 Lakeside Dr. Lynchburg, VA 24501, USA
* Corresponding author. Department of Obstetrics and Gynecology, University of Colorado Anschutz Campus, Mail stop B198-2 Academic Office 1 12631 East, 17th Avenue, Room. 4-2111 Aurora, CO 80045.
E-mail address: kweikelpa@gmail.com

Physician Assist Clin 7 (2022) 513–520
https://doi.org/10.1016/j.cpha.2022.02.008
2405-7991/22/© 2022 Elsevier Inc. All rights reserved.

CLINICAL CASE

A 33-year-old G2P1 female presents to the outpatient OBGYN office for evaluation of first trimester vaginal bleeding at approximately 7 weeks' gestation based on her last menstrual period. Transvaginal ultrasound revealed no evidence of gestational sac or fetal pole in the uterus. There was a substantial amount of spongy-appearing tissue with small cystic structures observed within the endometrial cavity. There was no fluid in the cul-de-sac. Ovaries appeared within normal limits with small follicles bilaterally. Initial serum beta human chorionic gonadotropin (hCG) was greater than 200,000 mIU/mL. Based on these findings, molar pregnancy was suspected. After receiving informed consent, the patient underwent suction dilation and curettage the next day. Initial suspicion of molar pregnancy was confirmed by pathology which demonstrated enlarged hydropic villa with cistern formation and marked trophoblastic proliferation. Further evaluation of the cytotrophoblast cells revealed diploid DNA. The final diagnosis was a complete hydatidiform mole.

GESTATIONAL TROPHOBLASTIC DISEASE

A complete hydatidiform mole and a partial hydatidiform mole are the 2 distinct diagnoses that are generally referred to as GTD. They result from aberrant fertilization where there is an overabundance of paternal genetic material in comparison to maternal genetic material. Complete and partial molar pregnancies are characterized by their chromosomal configuration and histopathological makeup.[1] Risk factors for the development of a molar pregnancy include extremes of maternal age, history of spontaneous abortion, and history of previous molar pregnancy.[1,2]

COMPLETE HYDATIDIFORM MOLE
Chromosomal Make-Up

A complete mole is the result of the fertilization of a genetically void oocyte by 2 sperm or 1 sperm that duplicates chromosomes. The result is an overabundance of trophoblastic tissue with no fetal development. The most common chromosomal pattern is a 46, XX karyotype.[1] The incidence of a complete mole is 1 to 3 per 1000 pregnancies.[2]

Presentation

In the past, it was most common to diagnose a complete molar pregnancy in the second trimester.[3] In the second trimester, the most common presenting symptoms were excessive uterine size, vaginal bleeding often characterized by "grape-like" clots, hyperemesis, hyperthyroidism, and less commonly, respiratory failure.[3] With the advancement of ultrasound technology and the ability to monitor serum hCG levels, a diagnosis is most common in the first trimester even before clinical symptoms present. The most common clinical symptom presenting in 90% of cases is vaginal bleeding often between 6 and 16 weeks of gestation.[1] In addition, up to 15% of cases will present with bilateral theca lutein cyst enlargement of the ovaries.[1] Patients with a complete mole should also be evaluated for hyperthyroidism (**Box 1**). Although less common, some patients with complete moles may present with hyperemesis gravidarum and preeclampsia.[4]

Malignant Potential

It is more common for a complete mole to become invasive. Complete moles present a 15% risk of malignant change.[2] Please see the section on Gestational Trophoblastic Neoplasia for a brief overview.

Box 1
Laboratory evaluation of molar pregnancy[1,4]

1. *Serum hCG*—often greater than 100,000 mIU/mL in complete mole

2. *CBC*—to assess for anemia and assess the need to workup for possible coagulopathy

3. *CMP*—to assess liver and renal function; to evaluate for electrolyte disturbances if the patient has hyperemesis

4. *Thyroid function studies*—hyperthyroidism is common in complete mole; thyroid storm can occur in patients with hyperthyroidism or hCG levels greater than 500,000 mIU/mL

5. *Blood type*—Rh-negative patients will need to receive Rho(D) immunoglobulin

6. *Chest radiography*—recommended as initial modality over chest CT to evaluate for metastatic disease and staging

---

PARTIAL HYDATIDIFORM MOLE
Chromosomal Make-Up

Partial moles are the result of the fertilization of a normal ovum by 2 sperm. This results in a triploid karyotype, most commonly 69, XXY (**Table 1**).[1] The incidence of a partial mole is approximately 3 per 1000 pregnancies.[2] There is an overall 1% to 2% recurrence rate of molar pregnancy.[3] This presents about a 10 to 20 times increased risk than that of the general population.[1]

Presentation

Partial hydatidiform moles usually present with the symptoms of an incomplete or missed abortion. The most characteristic symptom is vaginal bleeding occurring in approximately 75% of patients.[1] Unlike patients with complete moles, patients with partial molar pregnancy usually present with uterine sizes that are normal or small for gestational age and hCG values are rarely greater than 100,000 mIU/mL.[1]

Malignant Potential

It is much more common for a complete mole to become invasive. However, for partial molar pregnancies, there is still a 0.5% to 1% risk of malignancy.[3]

DIAGNOSIS OF GESTATIONAL TROPHOBLASTIC DISEASE

A clinical diagnosis is established through presenting symptoms, laboratory findings, and ultrasound results. The recommended laboratories are outlined in Imaging **Box 1**. Definitive diagnosis is made after histopathological analysis of evacuated molar tissue, including the presence or absence of fetal tissue and chromosomal characteristics.

Imaging

Ultrasonography remains the main clinical diagnostic tool for molar pregnancies. Complete molar pregnancies are characterized on ultrasound by drastic swelling of the chorionic villi which reveals a vesicular pattern. In the first trimester, ultrasound findings may be less definitive. In these situations, an elevated serum hCG greater than 100,000 mIU/mL can help differentiate between a complete mole versus a missed abortion.[1]

Both partial and complete molar pregnancies have distinct findings on ultrasound and often both conditions can be identified in the first trimester. The main

Table 1
Histopathologic and clinical features of molar pregnancy[1–3]

	Histopathologic Features	Clinical Features
Partial Mole	Triploid karyotype (ie, 69, XXY) Abnormal fetal tissue Focal enlargement of villi Focal trophoblastic hyperplasia	Symptoms of incomplete or missed abortion Vaginal bleeding (75%) Normal or small uterine size for gestational age hCG rarely >100,000 mIU/mL
Complete Mole	Diploid karyotype (ie, 46, XX) No fetal tissue Drastic swelling of the chorionic villi Diffuse trophoblastic hyperplasia	Vaginal bleeding (90%) Theca lutein cyst enlargement of the ovaries Excessive uterine size hCG >100,000 mIU/mL

differentiating element is that partial moles include the presence of embryonic or fetal tissue. When ultrasonography of partial moles can visualize the presence of a fetus, the fetus often displays congenital abnormalities consistent with triploid karyotype and evidence of growth restriction. Congenital abnormalities include syndactyly and cleft lip. Another common finding on ultrasound includes focal cystic changes of villi and local hyperplasia of trophoblastic tissue.[1]

TREATMENT OF GESTATIONAL TROPHOBLASTIC DISEASE

For those patients who wish to preserve their reproductive function, suction dilation and curettage (D&C) is the mainstay of treatment. D&C enables the complete evacuation of molar tissue and reduces the risk of hemorrhage and infection. Patients with extremely high hCG levels and an enlarged uterus are at risk of developing respiratory distress, preeclampsia, and trophoblastic pulmonary emboli.[4] Patients who are Rh-negative should receive Rho(D) immunoglobulin at the time of the procedure.[1] For patients who do not desire future pregnancies, hysterectomy is an acceptable therapeutic option. Hysterectomy will eliminate the risk of locally invasive disease. However, it should be noted that even with hysterectomy metastatic disease can still be possible.[1] For this reason, it is vital to serially monitor serum hCG levels at the same laboratory after the evacuation of molar tissue. Serum hCG is monitored every 1 to 2 weeks until undetectable levels (<5 mIU/mL) are sustained for at least 3 weeks. After 3 weeks, some sources continue to monitor their patients monthly to ensure that the value remains undetectable for 6 months to 1 year.[1] Recurrent pregnancy would interfere with monitoring the hCG levels so patients should be educated about and provided with reliable contraception for at least 6 months to 1 year. For patients who are considered high risk following the evacuation of molar tissue (eg, complete molar pregnancy, sustained elevation in serial hCG, or patients with limited access to follow-up care), there is conflicting evidence on the use of prophylactic chemotherapy to prevent GTN. The 2 most common chemoprophylactic agents include methotrexate and actinomycin D. The decision to use chemoprophylaxis is made on a case-by-case basis and is beyond the scope of this article.[5]

GESTATIONAL TROPHOBLASTIC NEOPLASIA

GTN encompasses several distinct pathologies, including invasive mole (IM; previously referred to as chorioadenoma destruens), choriocarcinoma (CC), epitheloid trophoblastic tumor (ETT), and placental site trophoblastic tumor (PSTT). IMs can progress from partial or complete molar pregnancies but are more likely to occur in complete moles.[5] CCs often develop secondary to a molar pregnancy but can present after a spontaneous early pregnancy loss, an ectopic pregnancy, and even after an uncomplicated full-term gestation.[5]

INCIDENCE OF GESTATIONAL TROPHOBLASTIC NEOPLASIA

Most aberrant fertilizations resulting in GTD are molar pregnancies and of those abnormal pregnancies, approximately 50% will result in GTN.[5] Complete moles carry the highest risk of evolving into GTN.[5] Partial moles carry a risk of approximately 1%.[2] Approximately 25% of GTN cases occur in patients with a history of a recent ectopic pregnancy or spontaneous abortion and 25% occur after an otherwise normal term pregnancy. Approximately 15% of molar pregnancies are IMs, and about 5% are CCs.[6] Approximately 1% of GTNs are due to PSTTs and epithelioid trophoblastic tumors.[7] Placental site trophoblastic tumors, although rare, carry the highest mortality.[6] Placental site trophoblastic tumors and epithelioid trophoblastic tumors occur most often after pregnancies that are not molar and in otherwise uncomplicated pregnancies and term deliveries 95% of the time.[8]

PRESENTATION OF GESTATIONAL TROPHOBLASTIC NEOPLASIA

IMs usually present with abnormal uterine bleeding, pelvic and/or abdominal pain, uterus large for gestational age, theca luteal cysts, and abnormally elevated serum hCG levels.[5,8,9] CCs typically present with abnormal uterine bleeding, blue or purple vaginal nodules, an enlarged uterus, and very high serum hCG levels. Patients with metastatic disease may present with hemoptysis and cough, emesis, headaches, and hemorrhage. The risk of hemorrhage is high with CCs because of its ability to alter the endometrial vasculature. About 30% of patients will develop lung, liver, and brain metastases.[10] Epithelioid trophoblastic tumors and PSTTs present with abnormal uterine bleeding.

EVALUATION OF GESTATIONAL TROPHOBLASTIC NEOPLASIA

Patients with suspected GTN should have a complete history and physical examination. Lesions that can be visualized on pelvic examination should not be biopsied as there is a likelihood of uncontrolled bleeding.[9] Evaluation for metastatic disease includes chest radiography and computed tomography (CT) with contrast imaging of the pelvis and abdomen as the most common sites of metastases are the lung and liver.[10] CT evaluation of the chest may also be considered. MRI of the brain is preferred over CT unless pulmonary metastases are evident.[9,11]

Box 2
FIGO anatomic staging[11]

Stage I: Disease confined to the uterus

Stage II: Disease extends outside of the uterus, but is limited to the genital structures (adnexa, vagina, broad ligament)

Stage III: Disease extends to the lungs, with or without known genital tract involvement

Stage IV: All other metastatic sites

Table 2
Modified WHO prognostic scoring system as adapted by FIGO[12,13]

Scores	0	1	3	4
Age	< 40 y	≥ 40 y	–	–
Previous pregnancy	Molar	Abortion	Term	–
Months post pregnancy	< 4 mo	4 - <7 mo	7 - <13 mo	≥ 13 mo
Serum βhCG pretreatment (IU/L)	$< 10^3$	$10^3 - < 10^4$	$10^4 - < 10^5$	$\geq 10^5$
Largest tumor size	–	3 - <5 cm	≥ 5 cm	–
Sites of metastases	Pulmonary	Spleen, renal	Gastrointestinal	Hepatic, brain
Number of metastases	–	1–4	5–8	> 8
Hx failed chemotherapy	–	–	Single agent	≥ 2 agents

DIAGNOSIS OF GESTATIONAL TROPHOBLASTIC NEOPLASIA

The International Federation of Gynecology and Obstetrics (FIGO) developed criteria for diagnosing GTN. Criteria include using hCG levels over time and via histopathology for CC, PSTT, and ETT.[10]

In postmolar pregnancies, GTN can be diagnosed under the following circumstances:

When hCG plateaus and persists for 3 or more weeks; when hCG rises weekly for 2 or more weeks; when hCG remains elevated for 6 or more months; or by a histologic diagnosis based on pathology.[10,12] Once diagnosed, patients are referred to gynecologic oncology.

When patients are stratified by the FIGO and the World Health Organization (WHO) staging systems, approximately 81% of patients will have low-risk disease and approximately 18% will have high-risk disease.[6] Patients with low-risk disease will usually receive methotrexate unless resistance develops; in those cases, patients receive actinomycin-D.[10] The treatment of high-risk disease involves myriad chemotherapeutic regimens and is beyond the scope of this article; however, patients with epithelioid trophoblastic tumors and PSTTs should undergo hysterectomy due to significant risk of resistance to chemotherapy.[4] The FIGO and WHO staging systems are outlined in **Box 2** and **Table 2**.

PATIENT EDUCATION

Survival rates for low-risk disease are almost 100% and over 90% for high-risk disease, primarily due to marked sensitivity to systemic chemotherapeutic regimens.[4,14] The risk of recurrence after 1 year is 1.2% in low-risk patients and 0.9% in high-risk patients.[15] As such, the utility of monitoring hCG after 1 year has been debated.[4] In the United Kingdom, clinical practice guidelines recommend hCG surveillance for 10 years.[15] Patients who did not undergo hysterectomy should use reliable contraception for the first year postdiagnosis and undergo monthly hCG testing. Patients who desire another pregnancy should wait at least 1 year before attempting conception. Patients and their providers should create a surveillance plan through shared decision making.

SUMMARY

Although a diagnosis of GTD or GTN can be alarming, successful treatment as defined by overall survival approaches 100%. However, prompt diagnosis and referral are essential. Patients should be counseled on contraception during the first 6 months to 1 year if the uterus remains intact, and hCG monitoring should continue for at least 1 year.

CLINICS CARE POINTS

- GTD results from aberrant fertilization and encompasses 2 distinct diagnoses characterized by their chromosomal configuration and histopathological makeup:
  1. Complete hydatidiform mole
  2. Partial hydatidiform mole

- GTD is most commonly diagnosed in the first trimester of pregnancy based on elevated serum hCG and ultrasound findings. GTD commonly presents with vaginal bleeding. Complete moles are characterized by a uterus that is large for gestational age while partial molar pregnancy presents with uterine sizes that are normal or small for gestational age. Patients with a complete molar pregnancy may also present in the second trimester with hyperemesis, hyperthyroidism, and less commonly, respiratory failure.

- The mainstay of treatment for GTD is complete evacuation of molar tissue via suction dilation and curettage or hysterectomy. Serial monitoring of serum hCG and avoidance of conception for 6 to 12 months is vital to ensure that GTD does not progress to invasive disease known as gestational trophoblastic neoplasia (GTN). It should be noted that complete hydatidiform moles present a greater risk of malignancy.

- GTN often presents with abnormal uterine bleeding, pelvic and/or abdominal pain, uterus large for gestational age, and theca luteal cysts.

- GTN is suspected after GTD if serial serum hCG remains stagnant or elevates after evacuation of molar tissue. GTN encompasses several distinct pathologies, including:
  1. Invasive mole
  2. Choriocarcinoma
  3. Epitheloid trophoblastic tumor
  4. Placental site trophoblastic tumor

- GTN is diagnosed and staged based on the FIGO and WHO systems. All patients diagnosed with GTN will be promptly referred to gynecologic oncology for treatment ± chemotherapy and for further surveillance.

DISCLOSURE

The authors have nothing to disclose.

REFERENCES

1. Lurain JR. Hydatidiform mole recognition and management: molar pregnancies may be associated with serious morbidity so prompt diagnosis, appropriate management, and follow-up are essential. Contemp OB/GYN 2019;64(3):12–7. Accessed September 26, 2020. https://www.contemporaryobgyn.net/view/hydatidiform-mole-recognition-and-management.
2. Candelier JJ. The hydatidiform mole. Cell Adhes Migration 2016;10(1–2):226–35. https://doi.org/10.1080/19336918.2015.1093275.
3. Heller DS. Update on the pathology of gestational trophoblastic disease. APMIS 2018;126(7):647–54.
4. Elias KM, Berkowitz RS, Horowitz NS. Continued hCG surveillance following chemotherapy for gestational trophoblastic neoplasia: When is enough enough? Gynecol Oncol 2019;155(1):1–2. https://doi.org/10.1016/j.ygyno.2019.09.006.

5. Ning F, Hou H, Morse AN, et al. Understanding and management of gestational trophoblastic disease. F1000Res 2019;8. https://doi.org/10.12688/f1000research.14953.1. pii: F1000 Faculty Rev-428.

6. Brown J, Naumann RW, Seckl MJ, et al. 15years of progress in gestational trophoblastic disease: Scoring, standardization, and salvage. Gynecol Oncol 2017; 144(1):200–7. https://doi.org/10.1016/j.ygyno.2016.08.330. Epub 2016 Oct 13.

7. Abu-Rustum NR, Yashar C, Bean S, et al. Gestational trophoblastic neoplasia, version 2.2019. National Comprehensive Cancer Network Clinical Practice Guidelines in Oncology. J Natl Compr Canc Netw 2019;17(11). https://doi.org/10.6004/jccn.2019.0053.

8. Mangili G, Lorusso D, Brown J, et al. Trophoblastic disease review for diagnosis and management: a joint report from the International Society for the Study of Trophoblastic Disease, European Organisation for the Treatment of Trophoblastic Disease, and the Gynecologic Cancer InterGroup. Int J Gynecol Cancer 2014;24: S109–16. https://doi.org/10.1097/IGC.0000000000000294 [PMID: 25341573.

9. Elias KM, Berkowitz RS, Horowitz NS. State-of-the-art workup and initial management of newly diagnosed molar pregnancy and postmolar gestational trophoblastic neoplasia. J Natl Compr Canc Netw 2019;17(11). https://doi.org/10.6004/jnccn.2019.7364.

10. Braga A, Mora P, de Melo AC, et al. Challenges in the diagnosis and treatment of gestational trophoblastic neoplasia worldwide. World J Clin Oncol 2019;10(2): 28–37.

11. Ngan HYS, Seckl MJ, Berkowitz RS, et al. Update on the diagnosis and management of gestational trophoblastic disease. Int J Gynecol Obstet 2018;143(Suppl 2):79–85.

12. Ngan H, Bender H, Benedet JL, et al. (FIGO Committee on Gynecologic Oncology). Gestational Trophoblastic Neoplasia, FIGO 2000 staging and classification. Int J Gynecol Obstet 2003;83(S1):175–7.

13. FIGO Committee on Gynecologic Oncology. Current FIGO staging for cancer of the vagina, fallopian tube, ovary, and gestational trophoblastic neoplasia. Int J Gynecol Obstet 2009;105(1):3–4.

14. Alifrangis C, Agarwal R, Short D, et al. EMA/CO for high-risk gestational trophoblastic neoplasia: good outcomes with induction low-dose etoposide-cisplatin and genetic analysis. J Clin Oncol 2013;Eli31:280–6.

15. Balachandran K, Salawu A, Ghorani E, et al. When to stop human chorionic gonadotrophin (hCG) surveillance after treatment with chemotherapy for gestational trophoblastic neoplasia (GTN): A national analysis on over 4,000 patients. Gynecol Oncol 2019;155.

Gestational Diabetes

Lynne Meccariello, PA-C, MPAS

KEYWORDS

- Gestational diabetes • Insulin resistance • Shoulder dystocia • Macrosomia
- Type II DM

KEY POINTS

- GDM is the most common medical complication in pregnancy.
- Treatment is key in mitigating maternal and neonatal risks of GDM.
- Defects in β-cell function combined with factors impeding insulin sensitivity contribute to maternal hyperglycemia.
- Maternal hyperglycemia can lead to fetal macrosomia and risk of shoulder dystocia and operative delivery.

BACKGROUND AND PREVALENCE

Gestational diabetes mellitus (GDM) is defined as glucose intolerance that occurs during pregnancy. Approximately 7% of pregnancies in the United States are affected by diabetes, and 86% of those cases are due to gestational diabetes.[1] The prevalence of gestational diabetes correlates with the prevalence of type II diabetes in certain ethnic populations and with the obesity rates in those groups. The ethnic groups known to have the highest rates of GDM are Hispanic, Black, Indigenous Americans, Asian, and Pacific Islanders.[2] The risk of gestational diabetes also increases with age, as it does in cases of type II DM. Women who deliver their first child at age greater than 35 years have been shown to have a greater than 2-fold risk of developing GDM. Women who are obese have more than twice the odds of developing GDM compared with women of normal weight.[3] Other risk factors include a family history of diabetes, diabetes in a previous pregnancy, past pregnancy complicated by fetal macrosomia, and a history of stillbirth.

GDM has been associated with both short-term and long-term consequences for both mother and fetus. Short-term maternal consequences include an increased risk of preeclampsia and an increased risk of operative delivery. Short-term fetal consequences include macrosomia, hyperbilirubinemia, and the need for neonatal intensive care unit (NICU) admission. Approximately 70% of women with gestational diabetes will develop type II DM within 22 to 28 years after pregnancy.[4] The offspring

Department of Quality and Patient Safety, New York Presbyterian, 21 Audubon Avenue, Room 301 D, New York, NY 10032, USA
E-mail addresses: mecca336@gmail.com; lym9006@nyp.org

Physician Assist Clin 7 (2022) 521–532
https://doi.org/10.1016/j.cpha.2022.02.009
2405-7991/22/© 2022 Elsevier Inc. All rights reserved.

of mothers with GDM have been shown to have a higher incidence of childhood and adult-onset obesity and diabetes, independent of genetic predisposition.[5,6]

SCREENING AND DIAGNOSIS

The purpose of screening for GDM is to help mitigate the maternal and fetal consequences associated with diabetes in pregnancy. Early intervention is key to optimizing outcomes. In the past, screening for risk of GDM involved focusing on past obstetric outcomes and a family history of diabetes. Unfortunately, this method of screening failed to identify approximately half of the patients with GDM. In 1973, O'Sullivan, and colleagues[7] proposed a screening method for patients who were considered high risk for diabetes. Patients were given a 50 g oral glucose load and blood was drawn 1 hour later to assess the level of glucose. This screening method is now used for all patients without preexisting diabetes and is the accepted screening approach that is used by approximately 95% of obstetric providers in the United States.[8]

Timing of screening for GDM depends on risk factors. The American Diabetes Association (ADA)[9] proposed a strategy of early pregnancy screening for women who are overweight or obese (body mass index [BMI] >25) and who have one or more of the following risk factors: sedentary lifestyle, first degree relative with diabetes, high-risk ethnic group, previous infant with birthweight greater than 4000 g, previous history of GDM, hypertension, hyperlipidemia, polycystic ovarian syndrome, a hemoglobin A1C greater than 5.7%, an elevated fasting blood glucose, a history of cardiovascular disease, or any condition associated with insulin resistance. If early screening is negative, patients are recommended to repeat screening between 24 and 28 weeks gestation.

Patients who do not have risk factors are recommended to be screened between 24 and 28 weeks gestation.[10] Cutoff values for the 1-hour screen range between 130 and 140 mg/dL, depending on the institution. Further research is needed to establish whether one cutoff value is more effective than others, and recommendations have been made for standardization.[11] One-hour glucose values greater than 200 mg/dL are generally considered to be diagnostic of GDM and preclude further screening.

In the United States, a 2-step approach to testing for GDM is accepted by most of the institutions and providers. Patients who screen positive after the 50 g test proceed to a 100 g oral glucose tolerance test (3-hour OGTT). Patients are directed to fast for at least 8 hours before testing. A fasting glucose level is drawn followed by administration of the 100 g glucose load. Blood is then drawn 1, 2, and 3 hours following the glucose load. At least 2 of 4 values must be elevated in order to be considered diagnostic of GDM.

Carpenter and Coustan[12] have established an alternative for abnormal values. The Carpenter- Coustan criteria are more inclusive and have a lower threshold for diagnosis, thus increasing the number of patients who require treatment. There has been debate over which criteria are most appropriate to use. There is no agreed-on single national standard for these criteria, and it is left to individual institutions to adopt what is suitable for their patient populations. Please see **Table 1** for a comparison.

A study[14] comparing perinatal outcomes in patients who were diagnosed with GDM using the NDDG criteria versus patients who were diagnosed using the Carpenter-Coustan criteria was undertaken. Of 4659 patients who screened positive for GDM, 1082 of those patients met NDDG criteria and 1542 met Carpenter-Coustan criteria. Cost-effectiveness of using the lower threshold criteria has yet to be determined.[14]

Table 1
National Diabetes Data Group versus Carpenter-Coustan gestational diabetes mellitus diagnostic criteria

Time	NDDG Criteria[13]	Carpenter-Coustan Criteria[12]
Fasting	< 105 mg/dL	< 95 mg/dL
1 h	< 190 mg/dL	< 180 mg/dL
2 h	< 165 mg/dL	< 155 mg/dL
3 h	< 145 mg/dL	< 140 mg/dL

PATHOPHYSIOLOGY OF GESTATIONAL DIABETES MELLITUS

In normal pregnancy, pancreatic beta cells undergo hypertrophy and hyperplasia to accommodate the metabolic needs of pregnancy and are able to secrete insulin in order to maintain normal glucose levels. In pregnancies complicated by GDM, the beta cells are unable to keep up with the metabolic demands of pregnancy.[15] This, combined with a reduced state of insulin sensitivity in pregnancy, results in physiologic hyperglycemia. In GDM, changes in glucose metabolism mirror those of type II diabetes, but with more insulin resistance and an increase in pancreatic beta-cell decompensation. In addition, placental hormones including estrogen, progesterone, leptin, cortisone, placental lactogen, and placental growth hormone help to promote insulin resistance as pregnancy progresses. This process results in increased production of endogenous glucose and breakdown of fat stores.[15] The result is elevated blood glucose levels. Glucose is easily transported across the placenta and acts as fuel for fetal growth.

Insulin resistance in pregnancy can be exacerbated by advanced maternal age, pre pregnancy overweight/obesity, and a sedentary lifestyle. GDM can be thought of as early stage type II DM that appears during pregnancy.[16]

Obesity is associated with an increased release of free fatty acids and secretion of adipose-specific proteins such as adiponectin, resistin, retinol-binding protein 4, and leptin. Macrophages are activated and work to worsen adipose tissue inflammation, further decreasing insulin sensitivity in muscle and liver cells. Chronic low-grade activation of plasma inflammatory and biomarkers during pregnancies complicated by GDM may play a role in development of type II DM by causing a decrease in insulin sensitivity.[17]

THE WHITE CLASSIFICATION SYSTEM

In 1949, Priscilla White reviewed 439 cases of diabetic pregnancies delivered at the same institution over 15 years.[18] This study included 5% of patients who were diagnosed as having diabetes after a glucose tolerance test performed during pregnancy. The remaining 95% of the patients likely had type I diabetes. She developed a classification system with the intention of determining possible causes and prevention of perinatal complications related to diabetes in pregnancy. The original classification system was intended for cases of pregestational diabetes.

A revised system was created in 1980 to include gestational diabetes as class A.[18] In 1986, the American College of Obstetricians and Gynecologists (ACOG) divided class A into 2 subcategories for GDM and is currently the accepted classification system. (Table 2).

Table 2
The White classification system

Class	Description 18
A1	Gestational diabetes, controlled with diet
A2	Gestational diabetes, insufficient control with diet, insulin required
B	Age of onset 20 y or older, duration <10 y, no vascular disease
C	Age of onset 10–19 y or duration 10–19 y; minimal vascular disease
D	Age of onset younger than 10 y, duration over 20 y, background retinopathy or hypertension
R	Proliferative retinopathy or vitreous hemorrhage
F	Nephropathy with greater than 500 mg/dL proteinuria
RF	Coexisting criteria for R and F
H	Clinically evident arteriosclerotic heart disease
T	Prior renal transplant

The usefulness of this classification system as a guideline for treating *gestational* diabetes has been questioned, as its original intention was for use in management of *pregestational* diabetes. In 1994, the updated ACOG Technical Bulletin noted that improvements in clinical management of gestational diabetes, such as regular fetal testing and metabolic care, have essentially rendered the White classification as less informative.[19] However, this classification system continues to be used and referenced in publications about diabetes in pregnancy.

COMPLICATIONS OF GESTATIONAL DIABETES MELLITUS MATERNAL COMPLICATIONS

Preeclampsia (PE) affects 2% to 8% of pregnancies in nondiabetic women.[20,21] PE risk is increased 2- to 4-fold in pregnancies complicated by type I and type II DM. PE is diagnosed in 15% to 20% of pregnancies complicated by type I DM and 10% to 14% of pregnancies with type II DM.[20,21] GDM also increases PE risk. In 2009, the German Perinatal Quality Registry conducted a retrospective review of 647,392 pregnancies to determine the association between GDM and PE and found that the odds of PE were increased among patients with GDM. They controlled factors such as age, parity, multifetal pregnancy, weight status, nationality, and pregnancy weight gain.[22] Similar reviews conducted in Canada and Sweden also confirmed that GDM is an independent risk factor for PE.[23,24]

Risk factors of PE overlap with risk factors identified for gestational and type II DM: prepregnancy obesity, advanced maternal age, multiparity, multiple pregnancy, and nonwhite race.[19] Insulin resistance is also suspected to play a role in the pathophysiology of PE. Women who develop PE during pregnancy have been shown to have more insulin resistance before pregnancy compared with women who are normotensive in pregnancy[25]; this is explained, in part, by the associated risk factors for PE and GDM. Prepregnancy obesity and gestational weight gain seem to play key roles in both. It is not known whether GDM and PE share a common etiologic pathway, but there are similar features found in both conditions, such as endothelial dysfunction, angiogenic imbalance, increased oxidative stress (eg, high free radicals), and high triglycerides.[26,27] PE may be associated with a prepregnancy susceptibility to cardiovascular disease, and poor placentation found in PE would lead to endothelial dysfunction and inflammation as evidenced by angiogenic imbalance, high free radicals, and high triglycerides.[28] Beta-cell dysfunction seen in GDM leads to hyperglycemia, which also causes endothelial damage and inflammation, leading researchers to postulate that insulin resistance could be the common trigger for both GDM and PE.[29] Further studies are needed to test these theories.

PE is well known to be strongly associated with preterm birth, small for gestational age, placental abruption, low Apgar scores, and cesarean delivery.[30] GDM is also strongly associated with increased rates of operative delivery. Maternal hyperglycemia and obesity have both been observed to be contributing factors of large for gestational age (LGA) and macrosomic fetuses, leading to a higher risk of shoulder dystocia at delivery.[31] The main negative outcome of pregnancy complicated by GDM is excessive fetal size; 1 in 8 women with GDM delivers an LGA infant due to glucose intolerance.[32] Prolonged first and second stages of labor are commonly associated with fetal macrosomia, increasing the rates of cesarean delivery due to failed labor progress and increased rates of maternal hemorrhage.

GDM and its risk factors are precursors to metabolic syndrome, including type II DM. These conditions are associated with insulin resistance, vascular dysfunction, and atherosclerosis later in life. A small case-control study in 2005 showed that patients with a history of GDM had higher levels of inflammatory biomarkers and peripheral vascular resistance at around 4 years post partum compared with patients without GDM.[33] In 2020 a British Medical Journal meta-analysis found that in populations of women with a history of GDM, the cumulative rate of subsequent type II DM was 16.46%, and those women have approximately a 10-fold higher risk of developing type II DM.[34]

FETAL AND NEONATAL COMPLICATIONS

In pregnancies complicated by GDM, higher glucose levels cross the placenta into the fetal circulation, which in turn triggers the fetal pancreas to secrete insulin. The resulting hyperinsulinemia creates an increase in fetal fat and protein stores, resulting in macrosomia.

Macrosomia is defined as a birthweight greater than or equal to 4000 g regardless of gestational age. LGA is defined as a birth weight greater than 90th percentile for a given gestational age.[35] Women with GDM have higher rates of LGA and macrosomic newborns. Studies have shown that GDM, obesity, and excess gestational weight gain are all associated with fetal macrosomia.[36–39]

In fetuses affected by GDM, body fat distribution differs from fetuses of nondiabetic mothers, with a higher concentration found in the upper torso and abdomen.[40] In fetuses of nondiabetics, body fat is generally more evenly distributed. This distinction is key in assessing risks of fetal shoulder dystocia at delivery. Shoulder dystocia is a vaginal delivery that requires additional maneuvers to facilitate delivery. Shoulder dystocia complicates approximately 0.5% to 1% of vaginal deliveries,[41] and risks include brachial plexus injury, clavicular and humeral fractures, perinatal asphyxia, and hypoxic-ischemic encephalopathy, leading to an increased need for NICU admission and prolonged length of stay.

Another neonatal condition associated with hyperinsulinemia is hypoglycemia at birth; this is due to the fetal response to maternal hyperglycemia that occurs in utero. After birth, the neonatal pancreas continues to secrete insulin, causing hypoglycemia, and this may lead to more concerning complications such as neurologic damage, resulting in seizures, developmental delay, and impaired mental function. Macrosomic neonates also have a higher oxygen demand, which causes an increase in erythropoiesis and eventually polycythemia. Hyperbilirubinemia and jaundice occur when this excess number of red blood cells breaks down. The treatment is NICU admission for phototherapy.[42]

Patients with GDM are thought to be at an increased risk of stillbirth or intrauterine fetal demise. A recent prospective study[43] included 455 stillbirth cases and found that 52% of cases of stillbirths that occurred over 37 weeks were patients with GDM. They were also more likely to have a hypertensive disorder, a higher BMI, and were older than 35 years.

TREATMENT

The goal of treating GDM is to minimize as many neonatal and maternal complications as possible by controlling maternal hyperglycemia; this is accomplished by monitoring dietary intake and balancing carbohydrates, fats, and proteins. Ideally, counseling by a diabetes educator should be made available. General dietary guidelines include dividing caloric intake among 3 meals and 2 snacks per day. ACOG 19 has recommended distributing calories between 40% carbohydrates, 40% healthy fats, and 20% protein. The ADA recommends similar dietary guidelines as for those with pregestational DM, with protein requirements as 15% to 20% of calories.[44] The Institute of Medicine recommends that 20% to 35% of calories be from healthy fat, and complex carbohydrates with lower glycemic indexes, which reduce the need for insulin and decrease postprandial hyperglycemia.[45]

Patients are instructed on self-glucose monitoring, with daily fasting and either 1- or 2-hour postprandial blood glucose, and are advised to keep a record of glucose levels. The goal of fasting blood sugars[45] is to remain less than 95 mg/dL. The cutoff for 1-hour postprandial glucose is less than 140 mg/dL and 2-hour postprandial is less than 120 mg/dL. If these criteria are not met after a 10- to 14-day trial on a diabetic diet, then pharmacologic therapy is indicated.

Insulin continues to be the treatment of choice, as it does not cross the placenta and is recommended by both the ADA and ACOG.[46]

The dosage of insulin is based on weight, gestational age, and timing of hyperglycemia. Generally, both intermediate-acting insulin, such as neutral protamine hagedorn (NPH), and short-acting insulin, such as aspart (NovoLog) or lispro (Humalog), are used. Short-acting insulins are taken before a meal. Depending on when hyperglycemia occurs will determine what type of insulin is required. If fasting glucose levels are elevated, nighttime NPH as a single dose would be indicated. Persistent postprandial hyperglycemia would require short-acting insulin such as Humalog.[1] Alternatively, patients can be placed on a daily regimen of divided doses of intermediate- and short-acting insulin throughout the day, based on a total dose of 0.7 to 1.0 units/kg.[1]

If circumstances preclude the use of insulin, metformin and glyburide (glibenclamide) are the next options. Both metformin and glyburide have been demonstrated to cross the placenta. They have not been adequately studied for possible long-term effects on the fetus/neonate.

Oral hypoglycemic agents have been reported to fail to adequately control hyperglycemia in about 25% of patients with GDM. Metformin seems to be safer in pregnancy than glyburide.[46,47] Glyburide has been associated with higher birth weight and neonatal hypoglycemia.[46,47] The initial dose of metformin is 500 mg orally taken at bedtime. The maximum daily dose is 2500 to 3000 mg during pregnancy. Glyburide is usually initiated with 2.5 mg daily, with a maximum of 10 mg per day in divided doses. Peak onset of glyburide is 2 to 3 hours, so its effect may not be reflective when checking 1- or 2-hour postprandial blood glucose.

FETAL SURVEILLANCE

Patients with GDM are recommended to undergo episodic fetal testing in the third trimester.[48,49] The goal of antepartum surveillance is to reduce the risk of stillbirth.

Generally, patients undergo weekly or twice-weekly testing, including a fetal nonstress test (NST) and biophysical profile (BPP) to determine fetal well-being. An NST assesses fetal autonomic neurologic function. The NST is determined to be reactive or nonreactive, and the monitoring period should be 20 minutes (please see chapter on Labor and Delivery for more information on NST). The BPP assesses amniotic fluid volume, fetal movements, fetal tone, and fetal breathing movements. Each element is assigned a score of 2 if present or 0 if not present. The BPP is performed for more than 30 minutes. A score of 8 is considered normal. A score of 6 is considered equivocal and requires further evaluation and monitoring for decision regarding delivery. A score of 4 or less is considered abnormal, and delivery is indicated.[49] In most cases, normal fetal testing is very reassuring.

Patients who are on pharmacologic therapy for GDM are recommended to begin antepartum testing at 32 weeks until delivery. Ideally, an ultrasound to calculate the estimated fetal weight should be performed in the third trimester to assess for LGA or macrosomia. Pregnancies with coexisting hypertensive disorders will require increased frequency of testing. Patients whose diabetes is well controlled on diet alone are not required to undergo fetal surveillance before 40 weeks gestation.

Daily fetal kick counts are also recommended by many obstetric providers. A decrease in maternal perception of fetal movement may precede fetal demise. The ideal number and duration of counts has yet to be defined; however, a few approaches[50–52] have been studied and seem to be acceptable and reliable. One method is to instruct the patient to lie on her side and count distinct movements up to 10 in a period of 2 hours. If 10 are counted, then fetal well-being is reassuring. Another method is to instruct the patient to count movements for 1 hour 3 times per week to establish baseline fetal activity. If subsequent counts equal the baseline, the fetal well-being is reassuring. If fewer counts are perceived with either approach, further antepartum surveillance is warranted.[50–52]

TIMING AND MODE OF DELIVERY

The recommendation for induction of labor is based on glycemic control and suspicion of LGA or macrosomia. Patients with well-controlled GDM may continue the pregnancy until 40 weeks 6 days but are recommended to undergo antepartum fetal surveillance. The risk of stillbirth increases significantly after 40 weeks gestation. Induction of labor carries an increased risk of cesarean delivery, postpartum hemorrhage, and shoulder dystocia, especially in cases where macrosomia is suspected.[53,54] Patients should be counseled about these risks before scheduling induction. Fetal indications must also be taken into consideration, as there is an increased risk of NICU admissions for respiratory distress and transitional tachypnea of the newborn, especially in neonates born via cesarean delivery. Ideally, delivery should occur greater than or equal to 37 weeks to ensure adequate fetal lung maturity.

A multicenter randomized controlled trial[55] of cesarean rates in patients with mild GDM was conducted. Induction and spontaneous labor were compared in women delivering over 37 weeks. Patients who had expectant management were also compared with the induction group.

Secondary analysis showed that induction before 40 weeks did not increase the cesarean delivery rate in their population, likely due to lower numbers of cases of fetal macrosomia. However, they found an increasing trend in cesarean delivery rate with increasing gestational age at term, and induction of labor was associated with higher rates of cesarean delivery after 40 weeks.

Many proposals have been made in favor of elective cesarean delivery to avoid potential adverse outcomes such as brachial plexus injury. Shoulder dystocia complicates approximately 1% of all vaginal deliveries and can result in transient or permanent injury to the neonate. At any given birth weight, diabetes increases the risk of shoulder dystocia by 2- to 3-fold.[56–58] However, most of the neonates with birth weights less than 4500 g born to diabetic mothers do not experience shoulder dystocia.[56–58] It should be mentioned that estimating fetal weight in the third trimester is variable in accuracy, and macrosomia as an indication for elective cesarean delivery would not be cost-effective when considering maternal risk and length of hospitalization.[59]

INTRAPARTUM MANAGEMENT

Glucose monitoring during labor is necessary in order to minimize the risk of neonatal hypoglycemia. The frequency of glucose monitoring in labor is based on glycemic control and if antenatal pharmacologic therapy was required. Patients who are diet-controlled, or A1 White classification, can have their glucose levels checked every 4 hours. Blood glucose levels that ranged between 60 and 120 mg/dL can result in fewer episodes of neonatal hypoglycemia compared with tighter control in labor, that is, hourly glucose monitoring with treatment of glucose levels lower than 60 mg/dL or greater than 100 mg/dL.[60] If blood glucose levels exceed 120 mg/dL, intrapartum insulin therapy should be considered.[60] If insulin treatment is initiated, blood glucose monitoring should be performed hourly and the infusion rate adjusted accordingly.

Insulin is given in an intravenous solution of 5% dextrose in 0.9% normal saline. If blood glucose levels exceed 180 mg/dL, then the intravenous solution can be changed to normal saline. Patients undergoing cesarean delivery may receive a one-time subcutaneous insulin dose immediately before delivery to ensure euglycemia.[61] Protocols for intrapartum glucose monitoring vary between institutions.

POSTPARTUM CONSIDERATIONS

Patients with GDM during pregnancy are at risk of developing type II DM later in life. Glucose intolerance that persists in the postpartum period is found in populations where there are associated risk factors, especially obesity. Both ACOG and the ADA recommend postpartum glucose testing for patients with GDM 6 to 12 weeks postpartum.[1,62] The current approach is for patients to undergo a 2-hour 75 g OGTT. A fasting blood glucose less than 100 mg/dL and a 2-hour postprandial glucose less than 140 mg/dL are considered normal. If the fasting glucose is greater than or equal to 126 mg/dL or the 2-hour postprandial is greater than or equal to 200 mg/dL, the patient is diagnosed with diabetes. If a patient has normal testing, both ACOG and the ADA recommend repeat testing at least every 3 years.[1] It should be noted that postpartum testing rates are approximately 35%.

Breastfeeding decreases the likelihood of postprandial hyperglycemia and may result in false-negative OGTT results.[62]

CLINICS CARE POINTS

- Taking a careful obstetric and family history is crucial in identifying patients at risk for GDM and its complications.

- Patients with a 1-hour glucose screen of 200 mg/dL or more should be treated for GDM and should forgo a 3-hour oral glucose tolerance test.

- Partnering with a nutritionist and diabetes educator is essential for patient education of GDM; adherence to a diabetic diet is the most challenging aspect for patients with GDM.

DISCLOSURE

The author has no commercial or financial conflicts of interest.

REFERENCES

1. ACOG Practice Bulletin No. 190: Gestational Diabetes Mellitus. Obstet Gynecol 2018;131(2):e49–64.
2. Caughey AB, Cheng YW, Stotland NE, et al. Maternal and paternal race/ethnicity are both associated with gestational diabetes. Am J Obstet Gynecol 2010;202(6): 616.e1–5.
3. Casagrande SS, Linder B, Cowie CC. Prevalence of gestational diabetes and subsequent Type 2 diabetes among U.S. Women. Diabetes Res Clin Pract 2018;141:200–8.
4. Kim C, Newton KM, Knopp RH. Gestational diabetes and the incidence of Type 2 diabetes: a systemic review. Diabetes Care 2002;25(10):1862–8.
5. Dabelea D, Hanson RL, Lindsay RS, et al. Intrauterine exposure to diabetes conveys risks for type 2 diabetes and obesity: a study of discordant sibships Diabetes 2000;49(12):2208–11.
6. Clausen TD, Mathiesen ER, Hansen T, et al. Overweight and the metabolic syndrome in adult offspring of women with diet-treated gestational diabetes mellitus or type 1 diabetes. J Clin Endocrinol Metab 2009;94(7):2464–70.
7. O' Sullivan JB, Mahan CM, Charles D, et al. Screening criteria for high-risk gestational diabetic patients. Am J Obstet Gynecol 1973;116(7):895–900.
8. Gabbe SG, Gregory RP, Power ML, et al. Management of diabetes mellitus by obstetrician-gynecologists. Obstet Gynecol 2004;103:1229–34.
9. American Diabetes Association. Classification and diagnosis of diabetes. Diabetes Care 2017;40(Suppl 1):S11–24.
10. Moyer V, U. S. Preventive Services Task Force. Screening for gestational diabetes mellitus: U.S. Preventive Services Task Force recommendation statement. Ann Intern Med 2014;160(6):414–20.
11. Vandorsten JP, Dodson WC, Espeland MA, et al. NIH consensus development conference: diagnosing gestational diabetes mellitus. NIH Consens State Sci Statements 2013;29(1):1–31.
12. Carpenter MW, Coustan DR. Criteria for screening tests for gestational diabetes. Am J Obstet Gynecol 1982;144:768–73.
13. National Diabetes Data Group. Classification and diagnosis of diabetes mellitus and other categories of glucose intolerance. Diabetes 1979;28:1039–57.
14. Beggren EK, Boggess KA, Stuebe AM, et al. National Diabetes Data Group vs Carpenter-Coustan criteria to diagnose gestational diabetes. Am J Obstet Gynecol 2011;205(3):253.e1–7.
15. Plows JF, Stanley JL, Baker PN, et al. The Pathophysiology of Gestational Diabetes Mellitus. Int J Mol Sci 2018;19(11):3342.
16. Chiefari E, Arcidiacono B, Foti D, et al. Gestational diabetes mellitus: an updated overview. J Endocrinol Invest 2017;40(9):899–909.

17. Abell SK, De Courten B, Boyle JA, et al. Inflammatory and other biomarkers: role in pathophysiology and prediction of gestational diabetes mellitus. Int J Mol Sci 2015;16(6):13442–73.
18. Sacks DA, Metzger BE. Classification of diabetes in pregnancy: time to reassess the alphabet. Obstet Gynecol 2013;121(2):345–8.
19. Obstet Gynecol Technical Bulletin 200. Diabetes in pregnancy. Washington (DC): ACOG; 1994.
20. Bryson CL, Ioannou GN, Rulyak SJ, et al. Association between gestational diabetes and pregnancy-induced hypertension. Am J Epidemiol 2003;158(12): 1148–53.
21. Knight KM, Thornburg LL, Pressman E. Pregnancy outcomes in type 2 diabetic patients as compared with type1 diabetic patients and non-diabetic controls. J Reprod Med 2012;57(9–10):397–404.
22. Schneider S, Freerksen N, Rohrig S, et al. Gestational diabetes and pre-eclampsia- similar risk factor profiles? Early Hum Dev 2012;88(3):179–84.
23. Nernenberg KA, Johnson JA, Leung B, et al. Risks of gestational diabetes and pre-eclampsia over the last decade in a cohort of Alberta women. J Obstet Gynaecol Can 2013;35(11):986–94.
24. Ostlund I, Haglund B, Hanson U. Gestational diabetes and pre-eclampsia. Eur J Obstet Gynecol Reprod Biol 2004;113(1):12–6.
25. Valdes E, Sepulveda-Martinez A, Manukian B, et al. Assessment of pregestational insulin resistance as a risk factor or preeclampsia. Gynecol Obstet Invest 2014; 77(2):111–6.
26. Zhou J, Zhao X, Wang Z, et al. Combination of lipids and uric acid in mid-second trimester can be used to predict adverse pregnancy outcomes. J Matern Fetal Neonatal Med 2012;25(12):2633–8.
27. Wizitzer A, Mayer A, Novack V, et al. Association of lipid levels during gestation with preeclampsia and gestational diabetes mellitus: a population-based study. Am J Obstet Gynecol 2009;201(5):482.el-8.
28. Wen SW, Xie RH, Tan H, et al. Preeclampsia and gestational diabetes mellitus: pre-conception origins? Med Hypotheses 2012;79(1):120–5.
29. Mastrogiannis DS, Spiliopoulos M, Mulla W, et al. Insulin Resistance: the possible link between gestational diabetes mellitus and hypertensive disorders of pregnancy. Curr Diab Rep 2009;9(4):296–302.
30. Shen M, Smith GN, Rodger M, et al. Comparison of risk factors and outcomes of gestational hypertension and pre-eclampsia. PLoS One 2017;12(4):e0175914.
31. Spellacy WN, Miller S, Winegar A, et al. Macrosomia-maternal characteristics and infant complications. Obstet Gynecol 1985;66:158–61.
32. Casey BM, Lucas MJ, Mcintire DD, et al. Pregnancy outcomes in women with gestational diabetes compared with the general obstetric population. Obstet Gynecol 1997;90(6):869–73.
33. Heitritter SM, Solomon CG, Mitchell GF, et al. Subclinical inflammation and vascular dysfunction in women with previous gestational diabetes mellitus. J Clin Endocrinol Metab 2005;90(7):3983–8.
34. Vounzoulaki E, Khunti K, Abner SC, et al. Progression to type 2 diabetes in women with a known history of gestational diabetes: systemic review and meta-analysis. BMJ 2020;369:m1361.
35. Macrosomia. ACOG Practice Bulletin Number 216; 135 (1) Jan 2020.
36. Black MH, Sacks DA, Xiang AH, et al. The relative contribution of pre-pregnancy overweight and obesity, gestational weight gain, and IADPSG-defined gestational diabetes to fetal overgrowth. Diabetes Care 2013;36(8):e128.

37. Alberico S, Montico M, Barresi V, et al. The role of gestational diabetes, pre-pregnancy body mass index and gestational weight gain on the risk of newborn macrosomia: results from a prospective multicenter study. BMC Pregnancy Childbirth 2014;14:23.

38. Bowers K, Laughon SK, Kiely M, et al. Gestational diabetes, pre-pregnancy obesity and pregnancy weight gain in relation to excess fetal growth: variations by race/ethnicity. Diabetologia 2013;56(6):1263–71.

39. HAPO Study Cooperative Research Group. Hyperglycemia and Adverse Pregnancy Outcome (HAPO) Study: associations with neonatal anthropometrics. Diabetes 2009;58(2):453–9.

40. Kamana K, Shakya S, Zhang H. Gestational diabetes mellitus and macrosomia: a literature review. Ann Nutr Metab 2015;66(Suppl 2):14–20.

41. Sentilhes L, Senat MV, Boulongne AI, et al. Shoulder dystocia: guidelines for clinical practice from the French College of Gynecologists and Obstetricians. Eur J Obstet Gynecol Reprod Biol 2016;203:156–61.

42. Riskin A, Itzchaki O, Bader D, et al. Perinatal outcomes in infants of mothers with diabetes in pregnancy. Isr Med Assoc J 2020;22(9):569–75.

43. Page JM, Allshouse AA, Cassimatis I, et al. Characteristics of Stillbirths associated with Diabetes in a Diverse U.S. Cohort. Obstet Gynecol 2020;136(6):1095–102.

44. Hernandez TL, Mande A, Barbour LA. Nutrition therapy within and beyond gestational diabetes. Diabetes Res Clin Pract 2018;145:39–50.

45. Landon MB, Spong CY, Thom E, et al. Anderson GB Eunice Kennedy Shriver National Institute of Child Health and Human Development Maternal-Fetal Medicine Units Network A multicenter, randomized trial of treatment for mild gestational diabetes. N Engl J Med 2009;361(14):1339–48.

46. Amin M, Suksomboon N, Poolsup N, et al. Comparison of glyburide with metformin in treating gestational diabetes mellitus: a systematic review and meta-analysis. Clin Drug Investig 2015;35:343–51.

47. Balsells M, Garcia-Patterson A, Sola I, et al. Glibenclamide, metformin and insulin for the treatment of gestational diabetes: a systematic review and meta-analysis. BMJ 2015;350:h102.

48. ACOG Committee Opinion Number 828 Indications for Outpatient Antepartum Surveillance. Obstet Gynecol June 2021;137(6):1148–51.

49. ACOG Practice Bulletin Number 229 Antepartum Fetal Surveillance-Interim update. Obstet Gynecol June 2021;137(6):e116–27.

50. Norman JE, Heazekkm AEP, Rodriguez A, et al. Awareness of fetal movements and care package to reduce fetal mortality (AFFIRM): a stepped wedge, cluster-randomized trial. AFFIRM investigators. Lancet 2018;392:1629–38.

51. Moore TR, Piacquadio K. A prospective evaluation of fetal movement screening to reduce the incidence of antepartum fetal death. Am J Obstet Gynecol 1989;160:1075–80.

52. Neldam S. Fetal movements as an indicator of fetal well-being. Dan Med Bull 1983;30:274–8.

53. Smith GC. Life-table analysis of the risk of perinatal death at term and post-term in singleton pregnancies. Am J Obstet Gynecol 2001;184:489–96.

54. Rand L, Robinson JN, Economy KE, et al. Post-term induction of labor revisited. Obstet Gynecol 2000;96:779–83.

55. Sutton AL, Mele L, Landon MB, et al. Delivery timing and cesarean delivery risk in women with mild gestational diabetes. Am J Obstet Gynecol 2014;211(3):244.e1-7.

56. Langer O, Berkus M, Huff RW, et al. Shoulder dystocia: Should the fetus weighing ≥ 4000grams be delivered by cesarean section? Am J Obstet Gynecol 1991;165: 831–7.

57. Lipscomb KR, Gregory K, Shaw K. The outcome of macrosomic infants weighting at least 4500grams: Los Angeles County and University of Southern California experience. Obstet Gynecol 1995;85:558–64.

58. Keller JD, Lopez-Zeno JA, Dooley DI, et al. Shoulder dystocia and birth trauma in gestational diabetes: a five-year experience. Am J Obstet Gynecol 1991;165: 928–30.

59. Rouse DJ, Owen J. Prophylactic cesarean delivery for fetal macrosomia diagnosed by means of ultrasonography- A Faustian bargain? Am J Obstet Gynecol 1999;181:332–8.

60. Hamel MS, Kanno LM, Has P, et al. Intrapartum glucose management in women with gestational diabetes mellitus: a randomized controlled trial. Obstet Gynecol 2019;133:1171–7.

61. Lende M, Rijhsinghani A. Gestational diabetes: overview with emphasis on medical management. Intern J Environ Res Public Health 2020;17:9573.

62. Carson MP, Cande VA, Gyamfi-Bannerman C, et al. Postpartum testing to detect persistent dysglycemia in women with gestational diabetes mellitus. Obstet Gynecol 2018;132(1):193–8.

Hypertensive Disorders of Pregnancy

Elijah A.J. Salzer, DMSc, PA-C, NYSAFE, C-EFM[a,b],*

KEYWORDS

- Gestational hypertension • Preeclampsia • Preeclampsia with severe features

KEY POINTS

- Hypertensive disorders of pregnancy (HDP) occur in up to 10% of all pregnancies and cause up to 16% of all maternal deaths.
- Neonatal complications include perinatal death and low birth weight.
- These syndromes include chronic hypertension, gestational hypertension, preeclampsia, superimposed preeclampsia, preeclampsia with severe features, eclampsia, and postpartum hypertension.
- Patients with a history of a hypertensive disorder are at significantly increased risk of developing cardiovascular disease later in life.

INTRODUCTION

Hippocrates of Kos is believed to have described eclampsia for the first time in fifth century BCE (εκλαμψια, translated as "a shining forth, exceeding brightness," probably from the older term, εκλαμπο, meaning "I burst forward violently"); in so doing, he wrote that "in pregnancy, drowsiness and headache accompanied by heaviness and convulsions is generally bad."[1] At present, the hypertensive disorders of pregnancy (HDPs) (chronic hypertension, gestational hypertension, preeclampsia, preeclampsia that is superimposed on chronic hypertension, preeclampsia with severe features, and postpartum hypertension) affect up to 10% of all pregnancies and are implicated in approximately 16% of maternal deaths.[2] Neonates delivered to patients with HDPs are at risk of perinatal death and low birth weight.[3] Between 1993 and 2014, these disorders increased in incidence in US women from 512 per 10,000 US women in 1993 to 912.4/10,000 in 2014.[4] Moreover, this entity results in death in non-Latinx black women at a rate 3 to 4 times that of non-Latinx white women.[5,6] In this article, the authors consider the 7 HDP-concerning risk factors, pathophysiology, definitions, symptoms, physical examination and laboratory findings, management, and prognosis.

a Department of Physician Assistant Studies, Pace University-Lenox Hill Hospital, 1 Pace Plaza, New York, NY 10038, USA; b Eastchester Medical Associates, P.C., Bronx, NY 10469, USA
* Corresponding author. Department of Physician Assistant Studies, Pace University-Lenox Hill Hospital, 1 Pace Plaza, New York, NY 10038.
E-mail address: esalzer@pace.edu

Physician Assist Clin 7 (2022) 533–544
https://doi.org/10.1016/j.cpha.2022.02.003
2405-7991/22/© 2022 Elsevier Inc. All rights reserved.

physicianassistant.theclinics.com

The HDPs include chronic hypertension, gestational hypertension, preeclampsia, superimposed preeclampsia, preeclampsia with severe features, eclampsia, and postpartum hypertension (**Table 1**).

PHYSIOLOGIC CHANGES OF PREGNANCY AFFECTING BLOOD PRESSURE

Some of the most dramatic changes in maternal physiology include those affecting the cardiovascular system, including an increase in blood volume of approximately 40% (and, of necessity, cardiac output). Primarily in the second trimester, peripheral vascular resistance is decreased due to effects from progesterone, nitric acid, prostaglandins, and arteriovenous shunting of blood to the uterus and placenta. This decreased resistance results in a relative reduction of mean arterial blood pressure (BP) until about 24 weeks' gestation. Despite an increase of renin and angiotensin II due to several factors, including placental production of estrogen,[8] most pregnant women are resistant to the increase in renin and angiotensin II.

PATHOPHYSIOLOGY OF HYPERTENSIVE DISORDERS

Numerous investigators have posited that preeclampsia can be divided into early- (occurring before 34 weeks gestational age) and late-onset preeclampsia (occurring at 34 weeks or thereafter) with placental abnormality noted more commonly in patients with early-onset preeclampsia, as was intrauterine growth restriction and stillbirth.[9,10] Maternal factors, such as obesity[7] and primiparity, were associated with late-onset preeclampsia.[11] Abnormal placentation is one cause of HDP.[12–15] Placentation involves in part the migration of cytotrophoblasts into the spiral arteries, causing changes within these vessels to increase blood flow. However, in patients who develop preeclampsia, pathologic changes that cause cytotrophoblasts to differentiate from a proliferative to an invasive type result in a narrowing of the spiral arterioles, placental ischemia, hypoxia,[16] and preeclampsia.[8,10] There is also an association between preeclampsia and third-trimester placental complications, including placenta accreta spectrum and retained placenta, suggesting a common pathway of these disorders.[9] The association between preeclampsia and autologous frozen embryo transfers or in donor oocyte recipient cycles in infertile patients may be due to in vitro fertilization,[17] increased serum estradiol levels, lack of relaxin production from the corpus luteum, ovarian hyperstimulation, or maternal immune response to paternally derived antigens.[18] Preeclampsia is also attributed to inhibition of vascular endothelial growth factor and placental growth factor by soluble fms-like tyrosine kinase 1 and thus causes an antiangiogenic effect.[19] Although preeclamptics have less circulating renin and angiotensin II compared with nonpreeclamptics, they have increased sensitivity to these hormones.[18]

Other risk factors for the HDPs are noted in **Table 2**.

CHRONIC HYPERTENSION

Approximately 10% of women of reproductive age are hypertensive.[20] In the context of pregnancy, chronic hypertension occurs before conception, to midpregnancy (20 weeks' gestation), or persists past 12 weeks after delivery. Chronic hypertension is defined by the International Society for the Study of Hypertension in Pregnancy (ISSHP) as the presence of systolic blood pressure (SBP) of at least 140 mm Hg and a diastolic BP (DBP) of at least 90 mm Hg on 2 separate occasions at least 4 hours apart.[21] However, although no changes in the definition are proposed at this time, Duffy and colleagues[22] have reported that a single elevated BP in gestation was

Table 1 Classification of hypertensive disorders of pregnancy[7]		
	Time of Diagnosis	Diagnostic Feature
Chronic hypertension	<20 wk	Hypertension ≥ 140/90 mm Hg present before conception or diagnosed <20 wk
Gestational hypertension	>20 wk	New-onset hypertension with the absence of proteinuria
Preeclampsia	>20 wk	New-onset hypertension and proteinuria (≥ 300 mg/24 h) or new-onset hypertension with end-organ dysfunction in the absence of proteinuria
Preeclampsia superimposed on chronic hypertension	>20 wk	Worsening hypertension with new onset of proteinuria or features of end-organ dysfunction

associated with the development of an HDP, abruptio placentae, cerebrovascular accident, and preterm delivery in a study of more than 300,000 gravid patients. Chronic hypertension in pregnancy is associated with superimposed preeclampsia, cesarean delivery, preterm delivery, low birth weight, and neonatal intensive care unit (NICU) admission.[23] The Fetal Medicine Foundation offers an online calculator to determine an individual patient's risk (https://www.fetalmedicine.org/research/assess/preeclampsia/first-trimester) **Box 1**.[24]

The management of chronic hypertension requires that the clinician be mindful of the benefit of lowered complications of pregnancy and of the risk of hypotensive episodes that could lead to other complications. The Control of Hypertension in Pregnancy Study (CHIPS) Trial defined "tight" BP control as a target DBP of 85 mm Hg and "less tight" control as a target DBP of 100 mm Hg. There was no difference in perinatal outcomes (perinatal death or admission to the NICU for >48 hours) between patients in the "tight" BP control group versus those in the "less tight" group; however, there was more severe hypertension seen in gravid patients in the "less tight" group.[25] Moreover, the ISSHP recommends "tight" BP control in patients with chronic hypertension.[26] **Table 3** lists the agents that may be used to control BP in nonurgent circumstances in patients with chronic hypertension.

GESTATIONAL HYPERTENSION

This condition that affects 5% to 10% of all pregnancies[27] is distinguished from chronic hypertension by the time during pregnancy when it presents, namely, at or after 20 weeks of gestation. Patients with gestational hypertension do not have a history of antecedent chronic hypertension. As with chronic hypertension, it is defined by the presence of SBP of at least 140 mm Hg and DBP of at least 90 mm Hg on 2 separate occasions at least 4 hours apart. Furthermore, none of the other conditions that define preeclampsia are present. Approximately 25% of patients with gestational hypertension will develop preeclampsia in the pregnancy; the earlier that the gestational hypertension presents, the higher the risk of preeclampsia.[21] As with preeclampsia, gestational hypertension confers on the patient an increased risk of cardiovascular disease later in life. Patients with gestational hypertension will require laboratory data listed in **Box 2** to rule out preeclampsia as well as close monitoring, including

Table 2
Risk factors for hypertensive disorders of pregnancy[2]

High-Risk Factors	Moderate-Risk Factors
History of preeclampsia, especially associated with adverse outcome	Nulliparity
Multifetal gestation	Obesity
Chronic hypertension	Family history of preeclampsia (mother or sister)
Pregestational diabetes	Demographic characteristics (African American or low socioeconomic status)
Renal disease	Age $\geq$ 35 y
Autoimmune disease	Personal history factors (ie, low-birth-weight infants, previous adverse pregnancy outcome, >10 y pregnancy interval)

BP at home and in the office. Medication is not indicated in the management of gestational hypertension alone.

Preeclampsia

Preeclampsia is a syndrome presenting at or after 20 weeks gestational age that includes hypertension accompanied by evidence of end-organ dysfunction affecting at least one of the following systems: renal, hepatic, hematologic, and/or the central nervous system. Symptoms may include severe headache, The BP parameters of preeclampsia are the same as that of chronic hypertension or gestational hypertension, for example, SBP greater than or equal to 140 mm Hg and/or DBP greater than or

Box 1
Suggested workup of women with chronic hypertension[18]

Explore lifestyle factors that could increase BP
   Assess excessive salt intake
   Assess excessive alcohol intake
   Sedentary lifestyle
   Medications or illicit substances that can increase BP (eg, decongestants, NSAIDs, immunosuppressants, antidepressants, cocaine)

Rule out obvious secondary causes of hypertension
   Serum electrolyte levels (including serum potassium and calcium levels)
   Serum creatinine level
   Thyroid-stimulating hormone
   Urinalysis

Evaluate baseline cardiovascular risk
   Fasting blood glucose level
   Lipid profile
   Electrocardiography

Establish results of baseline blood work critical to the evaluation of superimposed preeclampsia
   Complete blood cell count (particularly for platelet count)
   Serum creatinine levels
   Liver enzyme levels (AST or ALT)
   AST, alanine aminotransferase; AST, aspartate aminotransferase; NSAID, nonsteroidal anti-inflammatory drug.

equal to 90 mm Hg. In 2013, the American College of Obstetricians and Gynecologists Task Force on Hypertension and Pregnancy issued a report that updated definitions and management guidelines[28]; in 2018, the ISSHP updated its definitions and management guidelines. The criteria for evidence of end-organ dysfunction are given in **Table 4**.

Presentation of Preeclampsia

The patient may be asymptomatic or may present with a bilateral frontal or occipital headache that is often worse with an elevation of BP or with activity, and that does not improve with over-the-counter medications; indeed, headache due to preeclampsia is the most common cause of headache (other than tension headache or migraine headache) in pregnancy.[13] Patients may also present with dyspnea, visual changes, scotomata, and right upper quadrant and/or epigastric pain.[29] Although lower extremity edema is often seen in preeclamptic patients, it is no longer a diagnostic criterion.

Preeclampsia can be further subdivided between preeclampsia and preeclampsia with severe features. The difference between the 2 is that preeclampsia with severe features is defined by the presence of SBP of greater than or equal to 160 mm Hg and/or by DBP of greater than or equal to 110 mm Hg measured on 2 separate occasions 4 hours apart while the patient is at bed rest.[31] **Table 5** identifies the severe features of preeclampsia. The clinician should not be lulled into a false sense of security when managing the care of a patient with preeclampsia without severe features, as many acute syndromes in medicine, including the HDPs, can be unpredictable in their course and can worsen rapidly, with little warning.

HEMOLYSIS, ELEVATED LIVER ENZYMES, AND LOW PLATELETS

Although this life-threatening syndrome has been considered a complication of pre-eclampsia, up to 20% of patients with HELLP syndrome do not have a history of hypertension or other defining characteristics of preeclampsia at the time of the presentation of HELLP.[32] However, up to a fifth of preeclamptic patients will develop HELLP, and all patients with HELLP should be assumed to have preeclampsia.[25] Approximately 0.2% to 0.6% of all pregnancies will be associated with HELLP syndrome.[33]

Although patients may present with epigastric or right upper quadrant pain, headache, visual changes, and nausea and vomiting, this syndrome is diagnosed by the presence of hemolysis, elevated levels of transaminases, and thrombocytopenia and usually presents between 27 and 37 weeks of gestation.[34] Although **Table 6** notes the major diagnostic criteria for the 2 major classifications of HELLP syndrome, the reader should note that hemolysis is identified by schistocytes seen on peripheral smear, low serum haptoglobin levels, elevated indirect bilirubin levels, and elevated levels of lactate dehydrogenase.[32] Differential diagnosis of HELLP includes acute fatty liver of pregnancy as well as other thrombotic microangiopathies such as thrombotic thrombocytopenic purpura, and hemolytic-uremic syndrome[34]; it is also associated with the potential for disseminated intravascular coagulation (DIC)[32] and hematoma of the liver capsule.[35]

Management of HELLP syndrome is supportive. In pregnancies less than 24 weeks of gestation, termination is often recommended[36]; otherwise, antenatal steroids should be administered for pregnancies less than 34 weeks and magnesium sulfate for gestations less than 32 weeks to reduce neonatal morbidity.[32] Delivery is curative for HELLP syndrome, but the timing of delivery must be individualized. However, expeditious delivery should be undertaken in patients with severe, uncontrolled

Table 3
Suggested dose titration of antihypertensive therapy for nonurgent control of hypertension in pregnancy[18]

First Line	Low	If BP Not Controlled	Medium	If BP is Not Controlled on Medium Dosage	High	Maximum
Labetalol	100 mg tid–qid	Proceed to medium-dose of same low-dose medication	200 mg tid–qid	Consider adding another low-dose medication rather than going to a high dose of the same medication, for a maximum of 3 medications	300 mg tid–qid	1200 mg/d
Nifedipine (PA or MR)	10 mg po bid–tid		20 mg bid–tid		30 mg bid–tid	120 mg/d
Nifedipine (XL or LA)	30 mg qd		30 mg bid or 60 mg qd		30 mg qam and 60 mg qpm	120 mg/d
Methyldopa	250 mg tid–qid		500 mg tid–qid		750 mg tid	2500 mg/d

Abbreviations: bid, twice a day; LA, long acting; MR, modified release; PA, prolonged action; po, by mouth; qam, qd, every day; qid, 4 times a day; qpm; tid; 3 times a day; XL, extended release.

Box 2
Laboratory studies used in the diagnosis of preeclampsia

Complete blood cell count
Blood urea nitrogen
Creatinine
Transaminases
24-hour urine, or urine protein:creatinine ratio
Lactate dehydrogenase level
Uric acid level

---

hypertension, eclampsia, pulmonary edema, DIC, abnormal electronic fetal monitoring, abruptio placentae, or fetal demise.[37]

SUPERIMPOSED PREECLAMPSIA

This condition is defined as the development of preeclampsia in patients with an antecedent history of chronic hypertension. Approximately 26% of women with chronic hypertension will develop preeclampsia.[38]

PREECLAMPSIA WITH SEVERE FEATURES

This entity is distinguished from preeclampsia only by the presence of severe range BPs (SBP $\geq$ 160 mm Hg and/or DBP $\geq$ 110 mm Hg).

MANAGEMENT OF PREECLAMPSIA

All patients diagnosed with preeclampsia should be admitted to an antepartum unit.[24,39] If a patient is sufficiently stable for discharge, the patient should be seen by the clinician in the office twice a week for evaluation of repeat laboratory studies, physical examination, and review of BP readings. Ultrasound evaluation of the fetus (umbilical artery Doppler, measurement of amniotic fluid volume, and fetal measurements of biparietal diameter, head circumference, femur length, and abdominal circumference) should be evaluated weekly.[24] BPs should be maintained under "tight"

Table 4
International Society for the Study of Hypertension in Pregnancy 2018 definitions for preeclampsia[30]

Blood pressure	$\geq$ 140 mm Hg systolic and/or $\geq$ 90 mm Hg diastolic
Renal insufficiency	Creatinine >90 μmol/L, 1 mg/dL
Liver involvement	Elevated transaminases with or without right upper quadrant or epigastric abdominal pain
Neurologic complications	Eclampsia, altered mental status, blindness, stroke, hyperreflexia with clonus, severe headache with hyperreflexia, persistent visual scotomata
Hematologic complications	Thrombocytopenia with platelet count <150,000/dL, DIC, hemolysis
Uteroplacental dysfunction	Fetal growth restriction, abnormal umbilical artery Doppler wave

Abbreviation: DIC, disseminated intravascular coagulation.

Table 5
Severe features of preeclampsia[28]

Severe hypertension	SBP $\geq$ 160 mm Hg, DBP $\geq$ 110 mm Hg 2 Measurements 4 h apart at rest
CNS symptoms	Persistent headache Visual changes
Thrombocytopenia	Platelet count <100,000/mL
Renal insufficiency	Elevated creatinine level >1.1 mg/dL Doubling of baseline creatinine
Liver dysfunction	Levels of transaminases $\geq$ 2× upper limit of normal Persistent severe RUQ or epigastric tenderness
Pulmonary edema	Diagnosed on physical examination

Abbreviations: CNS, central nervous system; RUQ, right upper quadrant.

control as identified earlier with agents such as nifedipine, methyldopa, labetalol, oxprenolol, diltiazem, hydralazine, or prazosin.[24] When the patient is at 37 weeks' gestation, or if the clinical course worsens, the patient should be delivered.[26] Patients who are less than 34 weeks' gestation should be cared for under the supervision of a perinatologist. Indications for delivery for such patients include the inability to control BP; hypoxemia (oxygen saturation <90%); worsened transaminase values, hemolysis, creatinine values, and/or thrombocytopenia; continued or worsened neurologic symptoms or signs; eclampsia; evidence of abruptio placentae; reversed end-diastolic flow seen on umbilical artery Doppler; category 2 or 3 electronic fetal monitoring; or fetal demise.[24] Termination of pregnancy should be recommended at or before 24 weeks' gestation.[26]

Prophylaxis for eclampsia with magnesium sulfate ($MgSO_4$) should be used in patients with severe range BPs and neurologic symptoms[24]; any patient less than 32 weeks gestational age should also be given $MgSO_4$ for fetal neuroprotection, for example, to reduce the risk of cerebral palsy.[40] In either case, a loading dose of 4 to 6 g is given intravenously (IV), followed by 1 to 2 g/h via IV infusion. Fluid intake should be managed carefully to reduce the risk of pulmonary edema.

Table 6
Main diagnostic criteria for the Mississippi and Tennessee classifications of hemolysis, elevated liver enzymes, and low platelets syndrome[32]

	HELLP Class	Platelets (L)	AST[a] or ALT (IU/L)	LDH (IU/L)
Mississippi	1	$\leq$ 50 ×10^6	$\geq$ 70	$\geq$ 600
	2	$\leq$ 100 ×10^6– $\geq$ 50 ×10^6	$\geq$ 70	$\geq$ 600
	3	$\leq$ 150×10^6– $\geq$ 10 0×10^6	$\geq$ 40	$\geq$ 600
	Partial HELLP	Presence of 2 of the 3 aforementioned laboratory abnormalities along with evidence of severe preeclampsia or eclampsia		
Tennessee		$\leq$ 100 ×10^6	$\geq$ 70	$\geq$ 600

Abbreviations: ALT, alanine aminotransferase; AST, aspartate aminotransferase; LDH, lactate dehydrogenase.
[a] The Tennessee classification uses only AST readings.

Prevention of Preeclampsia

Through its effects on platelet aggregation and its effects on thromboxane A2, low-dose (80–100 mg daily) aspirin has been found to be of benefit in the prevention of preeclampsia, especially in patients who have a history significant for the disease.[41] Several meta-analyses of folic acid supplementation and reduction of the risk of preeclampsia[42–44] have not found a sufficient benefit to warrant its use at this time; further studies are needed. Several meta-analyses have reported a potential risk reduction of preeclampsia in patients taking calcium supplements during pregnancy.[45–47]

ECLAMPSIA

The most severe form of hypertensive disorders presents with tonic-clonic, focal, or multifocal seizures, often with a prodrome of severe frontal or occipital headache, visual changes, scotomata, or photophobia. Approximately 25% of cases do not present with hypertension or proteinuria and most cases occur during the antepartum course after 28 weeks' gestation.[48] Patients with eclampsia should be given magnesium sulfate 6 g IV over 15 to 20 minutes.[48] Delivery should be accomplished expeditiously. Maternal mortality may be as high as 7%, and the risk of perinatal mortality is as high as 11.8%.[48]

POSTPARTUM HYPERTENSION

Although usually preeclampsia is ultimately treated by delivery, up to 10% of recent parturients may present with an HDP during the puerperium.[49] The diagnostic criteria for this condition are an SBP of 150 mm Hg and a DBP of 100 mm Hg. Patients may also present with severe headache, blurred vision, scotomata, right upper quadrant or epigastric pain, dyspnea, and altered mental status in addition to the BP parameters noted earlier. BP normally decreases in the first 48 to 72 hours postpartum, so it is possible that this syndrome may not be recognized before discharge from the hospital. Most patients with HDPs will have clinical improvement within a week after delivery.[49] As part of its Safe Mother Initiative, the American College of Obstetricians and Gynecologists District II (New York State) has developed recommendations for patients with a history of preeclampsia that recommends BP measurement 72 hours after delivery with an outpatient evaluation within 3 to 5 days postpartum, repeated in 7 to 10 days postpartum or earlier if symptoms are present.[50] If SBP is persistently at or greater than 150 mm Hg or if DBP is persistently at or greater than 100 mm Hg, antihypertensive therapy is indicated with nifedipine, labetalol, captopril, or enalapril, all of which are considered to be safe in lactating patients.[49]

SUMMARY

The HDPs are common and can cause significant maternal and neonatal morbidity and mortality. With careful attention and management, complications can be reduced.

DISCLOSURE

The author has nothing to disclose.

REFERENCES

1. Lindheimer MD, Roberts JM, Cunningham FG, et al. Introduction, history, controversies, and definitions. In: Lindheimer MD, Roberts JM, editors. Cunning ham FC. Chesley's hypertensive disorders in pregnancy. . New York: Elsevier; 2000.

p. 1–23. Cited by: Rishniew M. Eclampsia in dogs: what's in a name? *Vet J* 2020;257:105437.

2. Sutton ALM, Harper LM, Tita ATN. Hypertensive disorders in pregnancy. Obstet Gynecol Clin North Am 2018;45:333–47.

3. Agrawal A, Wenger NK. Hypertension during pregnancy. *Curr Hypertens Rep* 2020;26:303–16.

4. Centers for Disease Control and Prevention. Data on selected pregnancy complications in the United States. Hypertensive disorders, 1993-2014. 2019. Available at: https://www.cdc.gov/reproductivehealth/maternalinfanthealth/pregnancy-complications-data.htm#hyper. Accessed June 27, 2021.

5. Hirshberg A, Srinivas SK. Epidemiology of maternal morbidity and mortality. Semin Perinatol 2017;41:332–7.

6. Zhang M, Wan P, Ng K, et al. Preeclampsia among African American pregnant women: an update on prevalence, complications, etiology, and biomarkers. Obstet Gynecol Surv 2020;75:111–20.

7. Shah S, Gupta A. Hypertensive disorders of pregnancy. Cardio Clin 2019;37: 345–54.

8. Irani RA, Xia Y. The functional role of the renin-angiotensin system in pregnancy and preeclampsia. Placenta 2008;29:763–71.

9. Wadhwani P, Saha PK, Kalra JK, et al. A study to compare maternal and perinatal outcomes of early vs. late onset preeclampsia. Obstet Gynecol Sci 2020;63: 270–7.

10. Bicocca MJ, Mendez-Figueroa H, Chauvan SP, et al. Maternal obesity and the risk of early-onset and late-onset hypertensive disorders of pregnancy. Obstet Gynecol 2020;136:118–127/.

11. You SH, Cheng PJ, Chung TT, et al. Population-based trends and risk factors of early- and late-onset preeclampsia in Taiwan 2001-2014. BMC Pregnancy Childbirth 2018;18:199.

12. Chau K, Hennessy A, Makris A. Placental growth factor and pre-eclampsia. J Hum Hypertens 2017;32:782–6.

13. Huppertz B. The critical role of abnormal trophoblast development in the etiology of preeclampsia. Curr Pharm Biotechnol 2018;19:771–80.

14. Ives CW, Sinkey R, Rajapreyar I, et al. Preeclampsia-pathophysiology and clinical presentations: JACC state-of-the-art review. J Am Coll Cardiol 2020;76:1690–702.

15. Rotem R, Pariente G, Golevski M, et al. Association between hypertensive disorders of pregnancy and third stage of labor placental complications. Pregnancy Hypertens 2018;13:166–70.

16. Nakashima A, Shima T, Tsuda S, et al. Disruption of placental homeostasis leads to preeclampsia. Int J Mol Sci 2020;21:3298.

17. Gui J, Ling Z, Hou X, et al. In vitro fertilization is associated with the onset and progression of preeclampsia. Placenta 2020;89:50–7.

18. Luke B, Brown MB, Eisenberg ML et al. In vitro fertilization and risk for hypertensive disorders of pregnancy: associations with treatment parameters. Am J Obstet Gynecol;2020:222:350.e1-350.e13.

19. Rana S, Lemoine E, Granger JP, et al. Preeclampsia: pathophysiology, challenges, and perspectives. Circ Res 2019;124:1094–112.

20. Battarbee AN, Sinkey RG, Harper LM, et al. Chronic hypertension in pregnancy. Am J Obstet Gynecol 2020;222:532–41.

21. Poon LC, Shennan A, Hyett JA, et al. The International Federation of Gynecology and Obstetrics (FIGO) initiative on pre-eclampsia: a pragmatic guide for first-

trimester screening and prevention. Int J Gynaecol Obstet 2019;145(Suppl 1):1–33.

22. Duffy JY, Getahun D, Chen Q, et al. Pregnancy outcomes associated with a single elevated blood pressure before 20 weeks gestation. Obstet Gynecol 2021;138: 42–50.

23. Magee LA, Khalil A, Kametas N, et al. Toward personalized management of chronic hypertension in pregnancy. Am J Obstet Gynecol 2020; S0002-9378(20):30745-6.

24. The Fetal Medicine Foundation. Risk assessment: risk for preeclampsia. Available at: https://fetalmedicine.org/research/assess/preeclampsia/first-trimester. Accessed July 20, 2021.

25. Magee LA, Rey E, Asztalos E, et al. Management of non-severe pregnancy hypertension -a summary of the CHIPS trial (Control of Hypertension in Pregnancy Study) research publications. Pregnancy Hypertens 2019;18:156–62.

26. Brown MA, Magee LA, Kenny LC, et al. Hypertensive disorders of pregnancy. ISSHP classification, diagnosis, and management recommendations for international practice. Hypertension 2018;72:24–43.

27. Shen M, Smith GN, Rodger M, et al. Comparison of risk factors and outcomes of gestational hypertension and pre-eclampsia. PLoS One 2017;12:e0175914.

28. American College of Obstetricians and Gynecologists. Task Force on Hypertension in Pregnancy. Hypertension in pregnancy. Report of the American College of Obstetricians and Gynecologists' Task Force on Hypertension in Pregnancy. Obstet Gynecol 2013;122:1122–31.

29. Wilkerson RG, Ogunbodede AC. Hypertensive disorders of pregnancy. Emerg Med Clin North Am 2019;37:301–16.

30. Bouter A, Duvekot JJ. Evaluation of the clinical impact of the revised ISSHP and ACOG definitions on preeclampsia. Pregnancy Hypertens 2020;19:206–11.

31. Other sources such as Magee, Rey, and Asztalos et al. report that the hypertensive criterion of pre-eclampsia with severe features may be observed when SBP of at least 160 mm Hg or DBP of at least 110 mm Hg that is then confirmed fifteen minutes later.24

32. Wallace C, Harris S, Addison A, et al. HELLP syndrome: pathophysiology and current therapies. Curr Pharm Biotechnol 2018;19:816–26.

33. Alese MO, Moodley J, Naicker T. Preeclampsia and HELLP syndrome, the role of the liver. J Matern Fetal Med 2021;34:117–23.

34. Szczepanski J, Griffin A, Novotny S, et al. Acute kidney injury in pregnancies complicated with preeclampsia or HELLP syndrome. Front Med 2020;7:1–11.

35. Fan H, Zhang P, Yang D, et al. HELLP syndrome complicated by subcapsular liver hematoma. Med Case Rep Study Protoc 2020;1:e0020.

36. Van Eerden L, Van Oostwaard MF, Zeeman GG, et al. Terminating pregnancy for severe hypertension when the fetus is considered non-viable: a retrospective cohort study. Eur J Obstet Gynecol Reprod Biol 2016;206:22–6.

37. Lam MTC, Dierking E. Intensive care unit issues in eclampsia and HELLP syndrome. Int J Crit Illn Inj Sci 2017;7:136–41.

38. Bramham K, Villa PM, Joslin JR, et al. Predisposition to superimposed pre-eclampsia in women with chronic hypertension: endothelial, renal, cardiac, and placental factors in a prospective longitudinal cohort. Hypertens Pregnancy 2020;39:326–35.

39. Ramos JGL, Sass N, Costa SHM. Preeclampsia Rev Bras Gineol Obstet 2017;39: 496–512.

40. Brookfield KF, Vinson A. Magnesium sulfate use for fetal neuroprotection. Curr Opin Obstet Gynecol 2019;31:110–5.
41. Atallah A, Lecarpentier E, Goffinet E, et al. Aspirin for prevention of preeclampsia. Drugs 2017;77:1819–31.
42. Liu C, Liu C, Wang Q, et al. Supplementation of folic acid in pregnancy and the risk of preeclampsia and gestational hypertension: a meta-analysis. Arch Gynecol Obstet 2018;298:697–704.
43. Hua X, Zhang J, Guo Y, et al. Effect of folic acid supplementation during pregnancy on gestational hypertension/preeclampsia: a systematic review and meta-analysis. Hypertens Pregnancy 2016;35:447–60.
44. Bulloch RE, Lovell AL, Jordan VMB, et al. Maternal folic acid supplementation for the prevention of preeclampsia: a systematic review and meta-analysis. Paediatr Perinat Epidemiol 2018;32:346–57.
45. Sun X, Li H, Xiyan He ML, et al. The association between calcium supplement and preeclampsia and gestational hypertension: a systematic review and meta-analysis of randomized trials. Hypertens Pregnancy 2019;38:129–39.
46. Hofmeyr GJ, Lawrie T, Atallah AN, et al. Calcium supplementation during pregnancy for preventing hypertensive disorders and related problems. Cochrane Database Syst Rev 2018;10:CD001059.
47. Khaing W, Vallibhakara SA-O, Tantrakul V, et al. Calcium and vitamin D supplementation for prevention of preeclampsia: a systematic review and network meta-analysis. Nutrients 2017;9:1141.
48. Bartal MF, Sibai BM. Eclampsia in the 21st century. Am J Obstet Gynecol 2022; 226(2S):S1237–353.
49. Katsi V, Skalis G, Vamvakou G, et al. Postpartum hypertension. Curr Hypertensive Rep 2020;22:58.
50. American College of Obstetricians and Gynecologists. District II. Safe motherhood initiative. Available at: https://www.acog.org/-/media/project/acog/acogorg/files/forms/districts/smi-hypertension-bundle-slides.pdf. Accessed July 26, 2021.

Placental Disorders

Elijah A.J. Salzer, DMSc, PA-C, NYSAFE, C-EFM[a,b,*]

KEYWORDS

- Placenta previa • Abruptio placentae • Placenta accreta spectrum • Vasa previa
- Subchorionic hemorrhage

KEY POINTS

- Common placental disorders include subchorionic hemorrhage, placenta previa, abruptio placentae, placenta accreta syndrome, single umbilical artery, and vasa previa.
- Except for single umbilical artery, these entities may present risks to the gravid patient, primarily those of hemorrhage, caesarean delivery, and at times, cesarean hysterectomy.
- In pregnancies affected by these conditions, the fetus is at risk of demise and complications of prematurity.

INTRODUCTION

The placenta is remarkable for being a temporary and mammalian organ created by the trophoblastic tissue that has already attached to the endometrium less than 2 weeks after ovulation.[1] In addition to being the largest fetal organ,[2] it sustains a dynamic, increasingly complex, and metabolically demanding fetus throughout approximately 280 days of gestation. The expulsion of placenta seems to decrease estrogen and progesterone production[3] and thus signifies the hormonal conclusion of pregnancy. Owing to various factors, including but not limited to infertility and its management, abnormal placental development, maternal age, parity, use of stimulants and tobacco, and trauma, a variety of conditions can occur that threaten the ability of the placenta to continue to support fetal development and survival.

PLACENTA PREVIA

Placenta previa (PP) is diagnosed when the placenta lies over the internal os of the cervix (**Fig. 1**). When the placenta is within 2 cm of the internal os, it is considered a low-lying placenta. Low-lying placenta remains one of the most feared obstetric complications due to its potential for causing maternal hemorrhage, which remains a significant cause of maternal morbidity and mortality.[5,6] This condition is increasing in incidence, largely because of the dramatic increase of cesarean deliveries, and is estimated to affect between 0.5% and 1.3% of all pregnancies[7,8]; in addition to its

[a] Department of Physician Assistant Studies, Pace University-Lenox Hill Hospital, 1 Pace Plaza, New York, NY 10038, USA; [b] Eastchester Medical Associates, P.C., Bronx, NY 10469, USA
* Corresponding author. Department of Physician Assistant Studies, Pace University-Lenox Hill Hospital, 1 Pace Plaza, New York, NY 10038.
E-mail address: esalzer@pace.edu

Physician Assist Clin 7 (2022) 545–557
https://doi.org/10.1016/j.cpha.2022.02.010
2405-7991/22/© 2022 Elsevier Inc. All rights reserved.
physicianassistant.theclinics.com

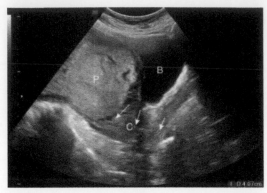

Fig. 1. Placenta previa.[4] (*From* Merriam A, D'Alton ME. "Placenta previa." In: In: Copel JA, D'Alton ME, Feltovich H et al. Obstetrical imaging: fetal diagnosis and care, 2nd ed. New York: Elsevier, 2018.)

association with hemorrhage, it is also associated with an increased risk of cesarean delivery, cesarean hysterectomy, succenturiate lobe, vasa previa (VP), prematurity, intrauterine growth restriction (IUGR),[9] and placenta accreta spectrum (PAS).[10] PP is believed to occur in patients with prior history of cesarean delivery primarily because of changes in blood flow within the endometrium and due to implantation of blastocysts in the vicinity of the scar.[7] Other factors that increase the risk of PP include advanced maternal age, higher-order parity, history of uterine instrumentation, infertility, and maternal use of stimulants and smoking.[11] Although the most common presentation is that of painless bright red bleeding in the third trimester, given the ubiquity of ultrasonography in developed nations today, most patients are diagnosed with PP via routine ultrasonography during the first or second trimesters. Clinicians must be mindful that approximately 66% to 98% of cases of PP and low-lying placentae are diagnosed before the third trimester; follow-up transvaginal ultrasonography should be obtained at 32 weeks.[12,13]

The use of transvaginal ultrasonography yields excellent sensitivity and specificity of the diagnosis of PP when compared with transabdominal ultrasonography.[9] Once the diagnosis has been made, outpatient management can usually be continued. However, patients with PP and other risk factors should be considered for admission. Patients at particular risk include those who live a significant distance from a tertiary care hospital with 24-hour obstetric anesthesia services or who have a concomitant history of antepartum hemorrhage, with short (<3 cm) cervical length, with a thick placental edge covering the internal os, or with history of prior cesarean delivery.[9] Bed rest is not recommended; the gravid patient may continue light exercise.[9] Although some authorities state that any vaginal or anal penetration be avoided (except for transvaginal ultrasonography),[9] others suggest that no evidence supports the avoidance of sexual relations that either do or do not result in orgasm in patients with PP.[14] Patients should be counseled about these modifications and should also be advised to seek immediate care in the case of bleeding or pelvic pain. Similarly, patients must be counseled about the need for cesarean delivery and of the potential for emergent delivery, blood transfusion, cesarean hysterectomy, prematurity, neonatal intensive care unit (NICU) admission, and maternal and fetal mortality.

In asymptomatic patients with confirmed PP with risk factors as noted earlier, cesarean delivery should be scheduled between 36 and 37 6/7 weeks gestational age (GA)[15]; those with a low-lying placenta within 1 cm of the internal os and with risk factors should be delivered via cesarean delivery between 37 and 37 6/7 weeks GA, and those with a low-lying placenta and without risk factors may be delivered between 38 and 38 6/7 weeks GA.[9] Antenatal corticosteroids should only be administered for fetal lung maturity to patients at very high risk of preterm delivery.[9]

PLACENTA ACCRETA SPECTRUM

PAS (**Fig. 2**) is the term used to describe placental invasion that extends through the endometrium, into or through the myometrium, into or through the serosa, or beyond, usually due to a uterine defect due to prior surgical or interventional radiologic procedures.[17] Such invasion may result in catastrophic bleeding requiring hysterectomy, blood transfusion, and other procedures. Previously, PAS was defined as 3 distinct conditions: placenta accreta, in which the chorionic villi contact the myometrium; placenta increta, in which the placenta invaded the myometrium; and placenta percreta, in which the villi have traversed the serosa.[18] However, today it is known as one spectrum disorder due to a lack of international agreement concerning the terminology.[19] The incidence of PAS has dramatically increased from roughly 1:4000 deliveries in the 1970s to as many as 1 in 500 deliveries in 2018,[20] probably because of the rapid and sustained increase in cesarean deliveries. Coexisting PP is also significantly associated with PAS; the risk is as high as 3% in women who have never had a previous cesarean delivery, and for patients with a history of 5 or more cesarean deliveries, the risk is 67%.[17] The risk is also increased in patients with prior history of uterine artery embolization, manual removal of the placenta, endometrial ablation, or hysteroscopic adhesiolysis.[4]

To reduce the risk of maternal and neonatal morbidity and mortality, it is ideal to diagnose PAS antenatally, if possible, via transvaginal ultrasonography[18,21]; such an approach also allows identifying placental location to rule in or out PP.[17] Although such studies are usually performed in the second or third trimester, it is at times possible to identify PAS in the first trimester via the findings of a gestational sac in the lower uterine segment, or lacunae identified in the placental bed.[19] In the second and third trimesters, increased placental vascularity noted via color Doppler, multiple vascular lacunae, and abnormalities of the interface between the bladder and uterine serosa are all findings suggestive of PAS.[17,22] MRI is considered to be equally accurate[20] as and not superior to ultrasonography[18] in diagnosing PAS. Consultation with a radiologist with particular expertise in PAS is warranted. Repeat imaging is recommended at 18 to 20, 28 to 30, and 32 to 34 weeks GA.[20] Patients must be counseled about the need for cesarean hysterectomy as well as the potential for blood transfusion, intensive care unit admission, deep vein thrombosis, NICU admission, prematurity, and maternal and neonatal mortality.

Up to 50% of patients with PAS will require transfusion, and 7% die of this syndrome.[23] Because of these and other risks, including that of disseminated intravascular coagulopathy and the need for multiple transfusions,[22] it is essential that patients with PAS are cared for in a level 3 or level 4 center to minimize morbidity and mortality for the parturient and neonate.[20] The care team should include specialists in gynecologic oncology, urology, urogynecology, interventional cardiology, perinatology, obstetric anesthesiology, neonatology, critical care, trauma, and vascular surgery.[18,20] Delivery should be accomplished via cesarean delivery, followed by a hysterectomy, between 34 and 35 6/7 weeks GA in asymptomatic patients; the uterus should be exteriorized after delivery with closure of the uterine incision and retention of the placenta to reduce the potential for significant bleeding.[20] The blood bank should be notified before surgery, if feasible, to permit preparation for massive transfusion.[18]

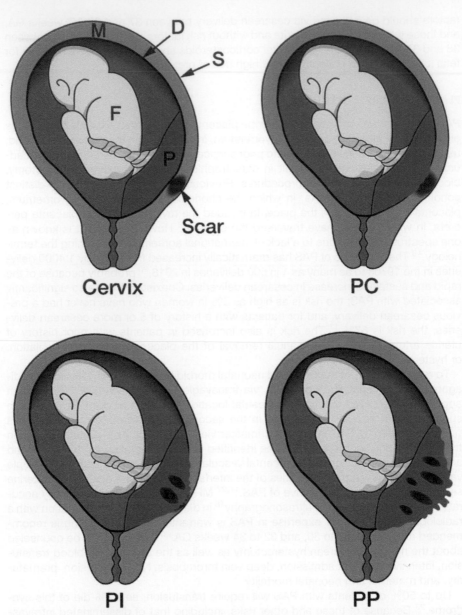

Fig. 2. Diagram showing normal and accreta placentation on a previous cesarean scar.[16] Anterior PP on a cesarean scar and different grades of PP accreta: creta where placenta villi adhere to myometrium without interposing decidual (D) tissue; increta where villi invade myometrium; and percreta where villi invade the entire myometrium and cross the uterine serosa. F, fetus; M, myometrium; P, placenta; PC, placenta creta; PI, placenta increta; PP, placenta percreta; S, serosa. Jauniaux E. Pathophysiology and ultrasound imaging of placenta accreta spectrum. Am J Obstet Gynecol 2018. (*From* Jauniaux E, Collins S, Burton GJ. Placenta accreta spectrum: pathophysiology and evidence-based anatomy for prenatal ultrasound imaging. Am J Obstet Gynecol 2018;218:75-87.)

ABRUPTIO PLACENTAE

Defined as the separation of the placenta from its uterine attachment after 20 weeks GA and before fetal delivery, this condition (**Fig. 3**) affects approximately 1% of all pregnancies[25] and results in perinatal mortality in approximately 10% of cases.[26] Abruptio placentae (AP) is the most common cause of bleeding after 20 weeks GA and most commonly occurs between 24 and 26 weeks GA.[27] In addition, AP can cause significant maternal morbidity, including antepartum or postpartum hemorrhage, sepsis, acute kidney injury, pulmonary edema, acute myocardial infarction, cardiomyopathy, disseminated intravascular coagulopathy death, and increased risk of transfusion and hysterectomy.[28,29] Neonatal complications include consequences of prematurity, hypoxia or asphyxia, IUGR, and congenital anomalies.[2,3]

AP most commonly occurs in patients who have had AP in a previous pregnancy. Other risk factors for AP include advanced maternal age, in vitro fertilization, thrombophilia, hypertension, preeclampsia, PP, chorioamnionitis, smoking, use of stimulants such as cocaine, trauma, multiple gestation, and African American race.[5,30-32] The pathophysiology of AP is uncertain but is believed to be due to abnormal trophoblastic invasion that leads to hemorrhage from the spiral arteries[33]; AP may be caused by an unknown event occurring early in pregnancy.[34] AP is diagnosed based on score on a scale of 0 to 3 in which 0 represents no symptoms with only a small retroplacental clot detected; 1 denotes vaginal bleeding, uterine irritability, and tenderness with no evidence of fetal or maternal distress; 2 is consistent with vaginal bleeding, uterine contractions, no signs of maternal shock, but with the presence of fetal distress; and 3 with evident or concealed severe bleeding, persistent abdominal pain, maternal shock, and fetal distress or death.[35]

Although the so-called classic presentation of AP includes dark red vaginal bleeding with passage of clots and tetanic uterine contractions, the accuracy of clinical findings alone is poor; one study found that only 38% of patients with AP had both pain and bleeding when diagnosed. One source reports that 35% fof present with occult abdominal bleeding, and 68% present with occult abdominal pain.[25] Patients may also present with decreased fetal movement, and cardiotocographic abnormalities are noted in most cases.[25] Obstetric ultrasonography demonstrates low sensitivity for AP.[36]

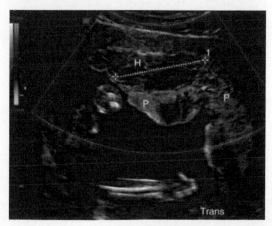

Fig. 3. Placental abruption.[24] (*From* Merriam A, D'Alton ME. "Placental abruption." In: Copel JA, D'Alton ME, Feltovich H et al. Obstetrical imaging: fetal diagnosis and care, 2nd ed. New York: Elsevier, 2018.)

Management of AP must first focus on maternal and fetal well-being. If the gravid patient is in shock, resuscitative measures must be undertaken expeditiously with large-bore intravenous (IV) access, IV fluids, and blood products. Once the mother is stabilized, plans for delivery will depend in part on the fetal status. In general, if the fetus is alive, emergent cesarean delivery is indicated; however, if there is fetal demise, vaginal delivery is preferable because it confers a lower risk of postpartum complications.[25] Aspirin greater than 100 mg daily instituted at or before 16 weeks GA may reduce the risk of AP in patients taking the drug for the prevention of preeclampsia.[37]

VASA PREVIA

VP (**Fig. 4**) is a rare entity affecting approximately 0.46 to 0.6 per 1000 pregnancies[39,40] that results from fetal vessels that are unprotected by Wharton jelly and that are placed through the membranes below the fetal presenting part and across the cervix.[41] VP either occurs when the vessel is connected to a velamentous cord

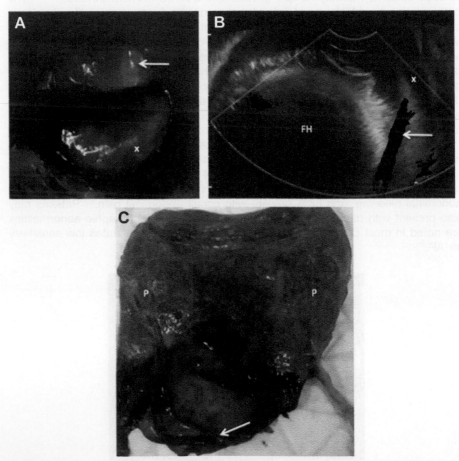

Fig. 4. Vasa previa[38] (*A*) amnioscopy showing vasa previa (*arrow*) in cervical dilatation area (X) (*B*) showing situation of vasa previa between fetal head (FH) and cervix (X) (*C*) showing two previa vessels connecting each part of bipartita placenta (P). (*From* Krief D, Naepels P, Chevreau J. Per labor vasa previa discovery: a simple clinical diagnosis. Eur J Obstet Gynecol reprod Biol 2018;231:284-285.)

(type I) or when it is instead connected with either a succenturiate or accessory placental lobe (type II).[4] These membranes can rupture and cause hemorrhage during spontaneous or artificial rupture of the membranes, or in the course of labor.[15] Because the fetal blood circulating volume is estimated to be less than or equal to 100 mL/kg, the fetus can exsanguinate rapidly[42,43]; when VP is not diagnosed antenatally, the risk of neonatal death is estimated at 60% or higher.[44] However, antenatal diagnosis and management can reduce this tragic statistic to nearly 0.[45]

Risk factors for VP include multiple gestation, velamentous cord insertion, presence of succenturiate lobe, and history of in vitro fertilization.[46] Clinically, VP should be suspected when a patient presents with painless vaginal bleeding, fetal distress, and rupture of the membranes.[47] However, today the diagnosis is usually made antenatally. Patients at high risk of VP, for example, those with a low-lying placenta, velamentous cord insertion, or succenturiate lobe should have a transvaginal ultrasonography with color Doppler; however, it is still possible for VP not to be identified with these modalities, and MRI remains an alternative to obstetric ultrasonography.[48]

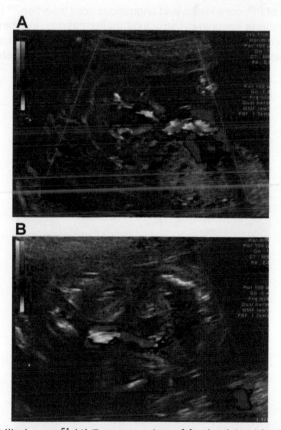

Fig. 5. Single umbilical artery[51] (A) Transverse view of fetal pelvis with color Doppler flow mapping showing bilateral umbilical arteries around the bladder in normal pregnancy (B) Transverse view of fetal pelvis with color Doppler ultrasound illustrating absence of color Doppler at the unilateral side of the umbilical artery in single umbilical artery. In this case, the right-side umbilical artery is missing. (From Wu Y-P, Tsai H-F, Cheng Y-C et al. Prenatal sonographic diagnosis of single umbilical artery: emphasis on the absent side and its relation to associated anomalies. Taiwan J Obstet Gynecol 2014;53:197-201.)

Patients diagnosed with VP antenatally should be considered for hospital admission at 30 to 32 weeks GA and should receive antenatal corticosteroids by 32 weeks; they should undergo scheduled cesarean delivery at 35 to 36 weeks, or emergently if spontaneous rupture of membranes occurs prior.[23]

SINGLE UMBILICAL ARTERY

The absence of 1 of the 2 umbilical arteries occurs in approximately 0.5% to 5% of pregnancies screened in the antenatal course,[49] in up to 1.6% euploid fetuses, but is more common in aneuploid fetuses, in which it is present in up to 11%.[50] Causes of single umbilical artery (SUA) (**Fig. 5**) include atrophy of a previously existing umbilical artery, primary agenesis, or persistence of the original allantoic artery of the body stalk.[52] Risk factors for this condition include advanced maternal age, smoking, multiple gestation, diabetes mellitus,[53] and in vitro fertilization. The term *isolated single umbilical artery* (iSUA) is used to denote cases in which there are no other fetal anomalies[54]; this entity is present in 80% of fetuses with SUA[55] and is also associated with an increased risk of PP, cord knots, and anomalous cord insertion.[56] In cases of SUA, fetal conditions include aneuploidy, structural malformations, low birth weight, NICU admission,[56,57] and IUGR,[58,59] with a higher incidence of such anomalies in cases of primary agenesis of the umbilical artery.[60] Thus, thorough anatomic scans are

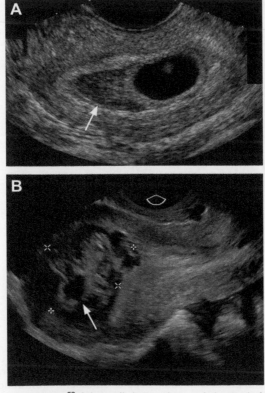

Fig. 6. Subchorionic hematoma[62] (*A*) Small, hypoechoic subchorionic bleed (less than one third of circumference of GS; *arrow*). (*B*) Large subchorionic bleed with heterogeneous echogenicity (between calipers) surrounding the GS (*arrow*). (*From* Mazzariol FS, Roberts J, Oh SK et al. Pearls and pitfalls in first-trimester obstetric sonography. Clin Imaging 2015;39:176-185.)

warranted when SUA is diagnosed during an obstetric ultrasonography in the mid-trimester. If iSUA is diagnosed, no other testing is indicated for aneuploidy.[61]

There is an increased risk of preterm birth, low birth weight, perinatal mortality, and hypertensive disorders in pregnancies affected by iSUA.[25,26] For fetuses with iSUA, the Society for Maternal-Fetal Medicine currently recommends a third-trimester ultra-sonography for growth and weekly fetal surveillance at 36 weeks GA.[61]

SUBCHORIONIC HEMATOMA

Approximately 25% of all pregnant patients will experience first-trimester vaginal bleeding; a subchorionic hematoma (ScH) (**Fig. 6**) is a common diagnosis made in the patient with such vaginal bleeding[63] and is also the most common sonographic anomaly detected in the first trimester in the presence of a live fetus.[64] The incidence ranges significantly between 0.46% and 39.5% of pregnancies.[65] The condition is identified ultrasonographically by a hypoechoic or anechoic, crescent-shaped area between the chorion and myometrium.[66] The mechanism of this lesion is unknown but is believed to be due to a partial detachment from the uterine wall by the chorion.[67] AP may develop from an ScH, in particular, if it occurs in a retroplacental area.[68] Assisted reproductive technology is considered a risk factor for ScH[69,70]; however, it is also possible that causes of infertility, such as uterine pathology, obesity, and others, are also factors.[71] Although a causal association has not yet been established, associations between ScH and spontaneous abortion, abruption, preterm prelabor rupture of membranes, IUGR, hypertensive disorders of pregnancy, and placenta previa have been found.[72] However, in the first trimester, it remains unclear whether ScH is a risk factor for pregnancy loss, and retroplacental hematoma seems to be more commonly associated with such losses.[54]

CLINICS CARE POINTS

- PP is associated with the potential for maternal hemorrhage, caesarean delivery, and caesarean hysterectomy.
- Most patients today are diagnosed with PP via routine obstetric ultrasonography before presenting with bleeding.
- PAS is associated with a history of concomitant PP and prior history of caesarean delivery as well as with a maternal mortality rate of 7%.
- AP is the most common cause of vaginal bleeding after 20 weeks of gestation and is associated with a history of hypertensive disorders of pregnancy, maternal trauma, smoking, amphetamine use, and leiomyomata uteri.
- VP occurs when fetal vessels not protected by Wharton jelly are placed through the membranes below the fetal presenting part and across the cervix.
- Isolated SUA is associated with an increased risk of preterm birth, low birth weight, perinatal mortality, and hypertensive disorders of pregnancy.
- ScH is a common diagnosis made in the patient with first-trimester vaginal bleeding and is also the most common sonographic anomaly detected in the first trimester in the presence of a live fetus.

DISCLOSURE

The author has nothing to disclose.

REFERENCES

1. Kurman RJ, Ellenson LH, Ronnett BM, editors. Blaustein's pathology of the female genital tract. 7th edition. New York: Springer; 2019. p. 1225.
2. Turco MY, Moffett A. Development of the human placenta. Development 2019; 146:dev163428.
3. Feinshtein V, Ben-Zvi Z, Sheiner E, et al. Progesterone levels in cesarean and normal delivered term placentas. Arch Gynecol Obstet 2010;281:387–92.
4. Merriam A, D'Alton ME. Placenta previa. In: Copel JA, D'Alton ME, Feltovich H, et al, editors. Obstetrical imaging: fetal diagnosis and care. 2nd edition. New York: Elsevier; 2018.
5. Sebghati M, Chandraharan E. An update on the risk factors for and management of obstetric haemorrhage. Womens Health 2017;13:34–40.
6. Fan D, Xia Q, Liu L, et al. The incidence of postpartum hemorrhage in pregnant women with placenta previa: a systematic review and meta-analysis. PLoS One 2017;12:e0170194.
7. Jauniaux E, Moffett A, Burton GJ. Placental implantation disorders. Obstet Gynecol Clin North Am 2020;47:117–32.
8. Gibbins KJ, Einerson BD, Varner MW, et al. Placenta previa and maternal hemorrhagic morbidity. J Maternl Fetal Neonatal Med 2018;31:494–9.
9. Babayla J, Desilets J, Shrem G. Placenta previa and the risk of intrauterine growth restriction (IUGR): a systematic review and meta-analysis. J Perinat Med 2019; 47:577–84.
10. Jain V, Bos H, Bujold E, Society of Obstetricians and Gynaecologists of Canada. SOGC clinical practice guideline: diagnosis and management of placenta previa. J Obstet Gynaecol Can 2020;42:906–17.
11. Grönvall M, Stefanovic V, Paavonen J, et al. Major or minor placenta previa: does it make a difference? Placenta 2019;85:9–14.
12. Durst JK, Tuuli MG, Temming LA, et al. Resolution of a low-lying placenta and placenta previa diagnosed at the midtrimester anatomy scan. J Ultrasound Med 2018;37:2011–9.
13. Reddy UM, Abuhamad AZ, Levin D, et al. Fetal imaging: executive summary. Am J Obstet Gynecol 2014;210(5):387–97.
14. McPhaedran SE. Sexual activity recommendations in high-risk pregnancies: what is the evidence? Sex Med Rev 2018;6:343–57.
15. American College of Obstetricians and Gynecologists. Medically indicated late-preterm and early-term deliveries. ACOG Committee Opinion #831. Washington, DC: ACOG; 2021.
16. Jauniaux E, Collins S, Burton GJ. Placenta accreta spectrum: pathophysiology and evidence-based anatomy for prenatal ultrasound imaging. Am J Obstet Gynecol 2018;218:75–87.
17. American College of Obstetricians and Gynecologists and the Society for Maternal-Fetal Medicine. Obstetric care consensus. Placenta accreta spectrum. Obstet Gynecol 2018;132:e259–75.
18. Garmi G, Salim R. Epidemiology, etiology, diagnosis, and management of placenta accreta. Obstet Gynecol Int 2012;2012:873929.
19. Berkley EM, Abuhamad A. imaging of placenta accreta spectrum. Clin Obstet Gynecol 2018;61:755–65.
20. Silver RM, Branch DW. Placenta accreta spectrum. N Eng J Med 2018;378: 1529–36.

21. Cal M, Ayres-de-Campos D, Jauniaux E. International survey of practices used in the diagnosis and management of placenta accreta specrum disorders. Int J Gynaecol Obstet 2018;140:307–11.

22. Cahill AG, Beigi R, Heine RP, et al, Wax JR for the Society of Gynecologic Oncology, the American College of Obstetricians and Gynecologists, and the Society for Maternal-Fetal Medicine. Placenta accreta spectrum. Am J Obstet Gynecol 2018;219:B2–16.

23. Silver RM. Abnormal placentation: placenta previa, vasa previa, and placenta accreta. Obstet Gynecol 2015;126:654–8.

24. Merriam A, D'Alton ME. Placental abruption. In: Copel JA, D'Alton ME, Feltovich H, et al, editors. Obstetrical imaging: fetal diagnosis and care. 2nd edition. New York: Elsevier; 2018.

25. Li Y, Tian Y, Liu N, et al. Analysis of 62 placental abruption cases. Risk factors and clinical outcomes. Taiwan J Obstet Gynecol 2019;58:223–6.

26. Riihimäki O, Metsäranta M, Paavonen J, et al. Placental abruption and child mortality. Pediatrics 2018;142:e20173915.

27. Kinoshita Toshihiko, Takeshita Naoki, Takashima Akiko, Yasuda Yutaka, Ishida Hiroaki, Manrai Megumi. A case of life-threatening obstetrical hemorrhage secondary to placental abruption at 17 weeks of gestation. Clinics and practice 2014;4(1):605.

28. Downes KL, Grantz KL, Shenassa ED. Maternal labor, delivery, and perinatal outcomes associated with placental abruption: a systematic review. Am J Perinatol 2017;34:935–57.

29. Elkafrawi D, Sisti G, Araji S, et al. Risk factors for neonatal/maternal morbidity and mortality in African American women with placental abruption. Medicina 2020;56:174.

30. Fadi SA, Linnau KF, Dihe MK. Placental abruption and hemorrhage-review of imaging appearance. Emerg Radiol 2019;26:87–97.

31. Tikkanen M, Nuutila M, Hillesmaa V, et al. Clinical presentation and risk factors of placental abruption. Acta Obstet Gynecol Scand 2006;85:700–5.

32. Huls CK, Detlefs C. Trauma in pregnancy. Semin Perinatol 2018;l42:13–20.

33. Bräila AD, Gluhovschi A, Neaçsu A, et al. Placental abruption: etiopathogenic aspects, diagnostic and therapeutic implications. Rom J Morphol Embryol 2018;58:187–95.

34. Elsasser DA, Ananth CV, Prasad V, et al. Diagnosis of placental abruption: relationship between clinical and histopathological findings. Eur J Obstet Gynecol Reprod Biol 2010;148:125.

35. Qiu Y, Wu L, Xiao Y, et al. Clinical analysis and classification of placental abruption. J Matern Fetal Neonatal Med 2021;34:2952–6.

36. Jha Priyanka, Melendres Giselle, Bijan Bijan, Ormsby Eleanor, Chu Lisa, Li Chin-Shang, McGahan John. Trauma in pregnant women: assessing detection of post-traumatic placental abruption on contrast-enhanced CT versus ultrasound. Abdom Radiol (NY) 2017;42(4):1062–7.

37. Roberge S, Bujold E, Nicolaides KH. Meta-analysis on the effect of aspirin use for prevention of preeclampsia on placental abruption and antepartum hemorrhage. Am J Obstet Gynecol 2018;218:483–9.

38. Krief D, Naepels P, Chevreau J. Per labor vasa previa discovery: a simple clinical diagnosis. Eur J Obstet Gynecol Reprod Biol 2018;231:284–5.

39. Westcott JM, Simpson S, Chasen S, et al. Prenatally diagnosed vasa previa: association with adverse obstetrical and neonatal outcomes. Am J Obstet Gynecol MFM 2020;2:100206.

40. Villani LA, Pavalaganthrajah S, D'Souza R. Variations in reported outcomes in studies on vasa previa: a systematic review. Am J Obstet Gynecol MFM 2020; 2:100116.
41. Melcer Y, Maymon R, Jauniaux E. Vasa previa: prenatal diagnosis and management. Curr Opin Obstet Gynecol 2018;30:385–91.
42. Swank ML, Garite TJ, Maurel K, et al. Vasa previa: diagnosis and management. Am J Obstet Gynecol 2016;215:223e1–6.
43. Fischel Bartal M, Sibai BM, Ilan H, et al. Prenatal diagnosis of vasa previa: outpatient versus inpatient management. Am J Perinatol 2019;36:422–7.
44. Jauniaux E, Silver RM. Rethinking prenatal screening for anomalies of placental and umbilical cord implantation. Obstet Gynecol 2020;136:1211–6.
45. Oyelese Y. Vasa previa: time to make a difference. Am J Obstet Gynecol 2019; 221:539–41.
46. Pavalagantarajah Sureka, Villani Linda, D'Souza Rohan. Vasa previa and associated risk factors: a systematic review and meta-analysis. American Journal of Obstetrics and Gynecology MFM 2020;2(3):100117. In press.
47. Derbala Y, Grochal F, Jeanty P. Vasa previa. J Prenat Med 2007;1:2–13.
48. Gagnon R. No. 231: guidelines for the management of vasa previa. J Obstet Gynaecol Can 2017;39:e415–21.
49. Li T-G, Wang G, Xie F, et al. Prenatal diagnosis of single umbilical artery and postpartum outcome. Eur J Obstet Gynecol Reprod Biol 2020;24:6–10.
50. Blum M, Weintraub AY, Baumfeld Y, et al. Perinatal outcomes of small for gestational age neonates born with an isolated single umbilical artery. Front Pediatr 2019;7:79.
51. Wu Y-P, Tsai H-F, Cheng Y-C, et al. Prenatal sonographic diagnosis of single umbilical artery: emphasis on the absent side and its relation to associated anomalies. Taiwan J Obstet Gynecol 2014;53:197–201.
52. Kim HJ, Kim J-H, Chay DB, et al. Association of isolated single umbilical artery with perinatal outcomes: systematic review and meta-analysis. Obstet Gynecol Sci 2017;60:266–73.
53. Gersell DJ, Kraus FT. Diseases of the placenta. In: Kurman RJ, Ellenson LH, Ronnett BM, editors. Blaustein's pathology of the female genital tract. 7th edition. New York: Springer; 2019.
54. Ebbing C, Kessler J, Moster D, et al. Isolated single umbilical artery and the risk of adverse perinatal outcome and third stage of labor complications: a population-based study. Acta Obstet Gynecol Scand 2020;99:374–80.
55. Li Tian-Gang, Guan Chong-Li, Wang Jian, Peng Mei-Juan. Comparative study of umbilical cord cross-sectional area in foetuses with isolated single umbilical artery and normal umbilical artery. Journal of Obstetrics and Gynaecology 2021;28:1–6.
56. Ebbing Cathrine, Kessler Jörg, Moster Dag, Rasmussen Svein. Isolated single umbilical artery and the risk of adverse perinatal outcome and third stage of labor complications: A population-based study. Acta Obstetrica et Gynecologica Scandinavica 2019;99(3):374–80.
57. Luo Xiaohua, Zhai Shanshan, Na Shi, Mei Li, Shishong Cui, Yajuan Xu, Limin Ran, Lidan Ren, Teng Hong, Rui Liu. The risk factors and neonatal outcomes of isolated single umbilical artery in singleton pregnancy: a meta-analysis. Scientific Reports 2017;7:7396.
58. Hua Meiling, Odibo Anthony, Macones George, Roehl Kimberly, Crane James, Cahill Alison. Single umbilical artery and its associated findings. Obstetrics and gynecology 2010;115(5):930–4.

59. Mailath-Pokorny Mariella, Worda Katharina, Schmid Maximilian, Polteraurer Stephan, Bettelheim Dieter. Isolated single umbilical artery: evaluating the risk of adverse pregnancy outcome. European Journal of Obstetrics, Gynecology, and Reproductive Biology 2015;184:80–3.

60. Hasegawa J. Ultrasound screening of umbilical cord abnormalities and delivery management. Placenta 2018;62:66–78.

61. Society for Maternal-Fetal Medicine. Society for Maternal-Fetal Medicine consult series #57: evaluation and management of isolated soft ultrasound markers for aneuploidy in the second trimester. (Replaces Consults #10, Single umbilical artery, October 2010; #16, Isolated echogenic bowel diagnosed on second-trimester ultrasound, August 2011; #17, Evaluation and management of isolated renal pelviectasis on second-trimester ultrasound, December 2011; #15, Isolated fetal choroid plexus cysts, April 2013; #27, Isolated echogenic intracardiac focus, August 2013). Am J Obstet Gynecol 2021;32. https://doi-org.eresources.mssm.edu/10.1016/j.ajog.2021.06.079.

62. Mazzariol FS, Roberts J, Oh SK, et al. Pearls and pitfalls in first-trimester obstetric sonography. Clin Imaging 2015;39:176–85.

63. Karaçor T, Bülbül M, Nacar MC, et al. The effect of vaginal bleeding and non-specific pelvic pain on pregnancy outcomes in subchorionic hematomas case. Ginekol Pol 2019;90:656–61.

64. Hashem A, Sarsam SD. The impact of incidental ultrasound finding of subchorionic and retroplacental hematoma in early pregnancy. J Obstet Gynecol India 2019;69:43–9.

65. Naert MN, Khadroui H, Rodriguez AM, et al. Association between first-trimester subchorionic hematomas and pregnancy loss in singleton pregnancies. Obstet Gynecol 2019;134:276–81.

66. Zhou J, Wu M, Wang B, et al. The effect of first trimester subchorionic hematoma on pregnancy outcomes in patients under went IVF/ICSI treatment. J Matern Fetal Neonatal Med 2017;30:406–10.

67. Sükür Yavuz, Göc Gösku, Köse Osman, Açmaz Gökhan, Özmen Batuhan, Atabekoglu Cem, Koç Acar, Söylemez Feride. The effects of subchorionic hematoma on pregnancy outcome in patients with threatened aboriton. Journal of Turkish-German Gynecological Association 2014;15(4):239–42.

68. Palatnik Anna, Grobman William. The relationship between first-trimester subchorionic hematoma, cervical length, and preterm birth. American Journal of Obstetrics and Gynecology 2015;213(3):403e1–4.

69. Reich J, Blakemore JK, Grifo JA. Comparison of subchorionic hematoma in medicated or natural single euploid frozen embryo transfer cycles. Fertil Steril 2020;114:595–600.

70. West BT, Kavoussi PK, Odenwald KC, et al. Factors associated with subchorionic hematoma formation in pregnancies achieved via assisted reproductive technologies. J Assist Reprod Genet 2020;37:305–9.

71. Rydze RT, Bosler J, Schoyer KD. Subchorionic hematoma and implantation: can better understanding the former help the latter? Fertil Steril 2020;114:509–10.

72. So S, Mochizuki O, Yamaguchi W, et al. Impact of subchorionic hematoma in early pregnancy on obstetric complications: a retrospective cohort study in women who had live births after frozen-thawed embryo transfer. Reprod Med Biol 2020;19:398–403.

Labor and Delivery

Melissa Rodriguez, DMSc, PA-C, FAAPA*,
Elyse Watkins, DHSc, PA-C, DFAAPA, NCMP

KEYWORDS

- Obstetrics • Gynecology • Labor • Delivery • Vaginal • Birth • Cesarean • Placenta

KEY POINTS

- The care of obstetric patients during the birthing process is innate and complex.
- Understanding normal physiology and abnormal situations are critical to responding to obstetric and neonatal emergencies.
- Evaluation of the pregnant patient in labor involves multiple components including the cervical examination, fetal heart tracing, and overall maternal-fetal status.
- Vaginal birth offers lower morbidity than cesarean delivery and should be the preferred method unless there is a medical or surgical indication.
- Management of labor, including induction and augmentation techniques, is important to facilitate a vaginal birth.

Abbreviations	
OBGYN	Obstetrics and Gynecology
PA	Physician Associate
ob	obstetrics
FHT	Fetal Heart Tracing

OBSTETRIC TRIAGE

The gateway to the labor and delivery unit is the obstetric (ob) triage, which can vary in size and capabilities depending on the institution. Often, the triage area consists of 3 to 6 rooms equipped with a gurney, a computer and monitor system, and an external fetal monitor. The external fetal monitor is used to assess the fetal heart rate (FHR) and uterine contraction pattern. There are also the necessary medical supplies such as gloves, lubricants, specula, and laboratory collection kits. Most triage bays will have an ultrasound machine with transabdominal and transvaginal

OBGYN PA, Department of Obstetrics and Gynecology, Advent Health Central Florida South Division, 380 Celebration Place, Celebration, FL 34747, USA
* Corresponding author.
E-mail address: merodriguez417@gmail.com
Twitter: @MelissaRodPA (M.R.)

Physician Assist Clin 7 (2022) 559–577
https://doi.org/10.1016/j.cpha.2022.02.004
physicianassistant.theclinics.com
2405-7991/22/© 2022 Elsevier Inc. All rights reserved.

probes for the evaluation of several maternal-fetal issues to be discussed later in this article. The most common chief complaints evaluated in the ob triage bay are contractions, possible rupture of membranes, vaginal bleeding, and decreased fetal movement. Other medical conditions may also be evaluated, including hypertension, asthma exacerbations, diabetes, and advanced maternal age. The most urgent conditions will be are listed in **Fig 1**.

Vaginal Bleeding

Many patients will experience bleeding during pregnancy, ranging from light spotting to a hemorrhage. The cervix is more vascular during pregnancy, and it is not uncommon to have some spotting after sexual intercourse, digital examinations, or pap tests. As the cervix dilates and effaces, patients may notice a "bloody show" consisting of light blood with intermixed cervical mucus. When presenting to the obstetric triage with vaginal bleeding during pregnancy, the evaluation will consist of a thorough history assessing the quantity of blood loss; possible infections; known abnormal placentation; recent intercourse or pelvic examinations; and any trauma, motor vehicle accidents (MVAs), or illicit drug use.[1] Physical examination will consist of a speculum examination to assess bleeding, cervical dilation, ectropion, cervicitis, and lacerations. Digital examinations are withheld until placenta previa has been ruled out. An ultrasound is performed to assess placentation, particularly if there is no previous documentation of placental location readily available. Rare conditions such as vasa previa, a condition where the umbilical vessels run through membranes covering the cervix, can lead to fetal distress, anemia, and demise. Therefore, this must be on the differential and rapidly ruled out.

Laboratory evaluation consists of a complete blood count, blood type, Rh status, and antibody screening. Coagulation factors, such as the partial thromboplastin time (PTT), prothrombin time (PT), and international normalized ratio (INR), are useful in identifying dysfunctions of coagulation. Elevated PT/INR and PTT are concerning for blood clotting inefficiency disorders (**Table 1**). Fibrinogen is elevated during pregnancy and is a useful test to monitor in cases of suspected placental abruption due to trauma, MVA, or illicit drug use, such as cocaine.

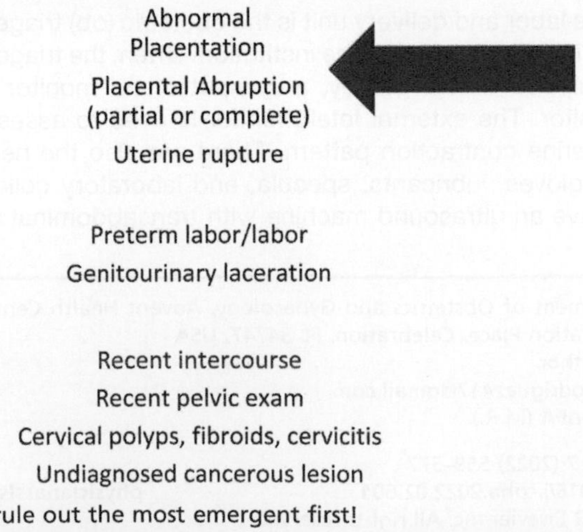

Abnormal
Placentation

Placental Abruption
(partial or complete)

Uterine rupture

Preterm labor/labor
Genitourinary laceration

Recent intercourse
Recent pelvic exam
Cervical polyps, fibroids, cervicitis
Undiagnosed cancerous lesion

Fig. 1. Urgency—rule out the most emergent first!

Table 1 Coagulation factors		
Laboratory	**Pathways**	**Uses**
PT/INR	Extrinsic system: a tissue factor produced from an injury interacts with factor VIIa to activate factor X to Xa common pathway	• Monitor medications • Diagnose coagulopathy • Prolonged = deficiency with factors VII, X, V, prothrombin, fibrinogen, vitamin K, liver disease, and those taking warfarin
aPTT	Intrinsic system: initiated by contact with a foreign substance and includes Factor XII ?Factor XIIa Factor XIIa + XI XIa Factor XIa + X Xa common pathway	• Diagnose bleeding disorders • Monitor anticlotting drugs, that is, heparin • Prolonged = missing or defective clotting factors, liver disease
Fibrinogen	Same as clotting factor I. Produced by the liver. Converted into insoluble fibrin by thrombin • Fibrinogen activity test evaluates function • *Fibrinogen antigen test evaluates amount (less common)*	• Diagnose bleeding disorder or inappropriate clot formation • Diagnose DIC where fibrinogen is consumed faster than it can be produced • Significantly decreased fibrinogen may be due to decreased amounts or decreased function

Abbreviations: aPTT, activated partial thromboplastin time; DIC, disseminated intravascular coagulation.

The management for vaginal bleeding will depend on the quantity and flow, gestational age, fetal status, maternal status, and relevant history, physical, laboratory, and imaging findings. For benign issues with normal maternal-fetal status, reassurance can be provided. Concerning situations will require prolonged observation in the unit. Worrisome or emergent conditions need to be addressed promptly.

Transfusion of blood products will depend on the maternal and fetal status, vital signs, laboratory findings, and quantification of the amount of blood lost. As noted in **Table 2**, the amount of blood volume lost usually correlates with the findings, and management is suggested based on the findings. The amount of any blood product can be determined based on the volumes per unit and determining how many units are needed to increase by a certain amount (**Table 3**).

Table 2 Blood loss volumes		
Blood Volume Loss		**Management**
Grade 1	15% (750 mL)	Normal vitals, no transfusion
Grade 2	15%–30% (750–1500 mL)	Crystalloids (3:1) or synthetic colloids
Grade 3	30%–40% (1500–2000 mL)	Crystalloids, blood products
Grade 4	≥40% (>2000 mL)	Crystalloids, PRBCs, PLT, FFP, cryoprecipitate

Abbreviations: FFP, fresh frozen plasma; PLT, platelet; PRBC, packed red blood cell.

Table 3 Blood products		
Blood Products		
PRBC	One pack = 250 mL	Increases HGB by 1 mg/dL Increases HCT by 3%
PLT	One unit = 6 packs	Increases PLT by 25,000–50,000
FFP	One unit = 200–250 mL Usually, 2–4 units given	Indication: bleeding and abnormal coagulation (INR > 1.5)
Cryoprecipitate	One unit = 15–20 mL Usually, 6 units given	Increases fibrinogen by 30–60 mg/dL per 6 units Indicated for fibrinogen < 100 (DIC)

Abbreviations: DIC, disseminated intravascular coagulation; FFP, fresh frozen plasma; PLT, platelet; PRBC, packed red blood cell; HGB, Hemoglobin; HCT, Hematocrit.

Decreased Fetal Movement

Fetal movement awareness is variable for each person. Typically, fetal movement counts begin at 28 weeks. Some underlying medical conditions warrant closer observation as they can cause fetal distress or demise. Always check for fetal cardiac activity as any delay in diagnosing a fetal demise is inappropriate and could be misconstrued as a delay in care. The first steps include placing an external fetal cardiac monitor to record heart tones as well as placement of a tocometer to assess contractions. Maternal vital signs are monitored simultaneously. Management depends on maternal and fetal status.

A reassuring fetal heart tracing is the ideal situation. Please refer to the section Electronic Fetal Monitoring for a more detailed description of various tracings. A biophysical profile can be performed to assess amniotic fluid, fetal movement, tone, and breathing (**Table 4**). Concerning situations will require prolonged monitoring and possible emergent or urgent intervention. Fetal demise is identified when there is absent cardiac activity on ultrasound and should be confirmed by 2 providers. Management of fetal demise will depend on the gestational age.

Ruptured Amniotic Membranes

Ruptured amniotic membranes can occur at any time during the pregnancy and the management depends on the gestational age of the fetus. See **Table 5** for a thorough explanation of rupture of membranes. Evaluation will always begin with a determination of whether amniotic fluid is present. Other causes of a chief complaint of "leaking"

Table 4 Biophysical profile	
Components	**Points are Either 0 or 2**
Amniotic fluid index	1 pocket >2 cm vertical measurement
Fetal tone	One or more episodes of extension and flexion of hands/limbs or trunk
Fetal movement	At least 3 discreet body/limb movements
Fetal breathing	One or more episodes of breathing for 30 s
NST	Two accelerations to meet reactivity criteria within 20 min

Abbreviations: NST, Non-Stress Test

Table 5
Rupture of membranes

ROM	Type	Management
PPROM	Preterm, <37 weeks' gestation	Collect GBS, UCS, GC/CT, routine laboratories Start antibiotics for latency if < 34 wk Assess for corticosteroids for fetal lung maturity based on guidelines If <32 weeks' gestation, start magnesium sulfate for neuroprotection Notify consultants (if applicable)
PROM	Term, Rupture onset before labor	Consider induction/augmentation of labor
SROM	Term, Rupture onset during labor	Continue routine management

Abbreviations: GBS, group B Streptococcus; GC/CT, gonorrhea and chlamydia; PPROM, preterm prelabor rupture of membranes; PROM, prelabor rupture of membranes; ROM rupture of membranes; SROM, spontaneous rupture of membrane; UCS, urine culture.

include urine and semen. A speculum examination is performed to assess for pooling of fluid in the posterior fornix of the vagina followed by the collection of fluid with a swab and smear on a glass slide to visualize under the microscope. A Ferning pattern occurs when the amniotic fluid crystallizes. Another test is to assess the pH level of the fluid with nitrazine paper. The more alkaline pH of amniotic fluid will turn the nitrazine test blue. However, bacteria, blood, and semen can also cause nitrazine to turn blue. Newer biochemical testing is available to assess for amniotic fluid leakage as well, including the ROMplus, which detects alpha-fetoprotein (AFP) and insulin-like growth factor-binding protein 1 (IGFBP-1) using a monoclonal/polyclonal antibody approach. Another test is called the AmniSure, which detects placental alpha-microglobulin-1 protein in vaginal fluid.

Preterm Labor

Preterm labor is the presence of cervical dilation and effacement before 36 weeks 6 days of gestation. Usually, patients will present with contractions and an accompanied cervical change, either dilation, effacement, or both. If an initial cervical dilation is at least 2 cm with regular uterine contractions, this diagnosis can also be made.[2] An additional tool is the use of transvaginal ultrasonography to assess the cervical length. With a shortened cervix, the risk for preterm delivery increases and is most predictive when found at less than 28 weeks' gestation. A cervical length less than or equal to 2 cm with regular uterine contractions is at high risk for preterm delivery within 7 days. If the cervical length is above 3 cm, there is a relatively low risk of preterm delivery within the next 7 days. Between 24 and 34 weeks' gestation, with a cervical dilation less than 3 cm, and a cervical length between 2 and 3 cm on transvaginal ultrasound, a fetal fibronectin test (fFN) can be performed to assess cervicovaginal secretions that occur with labor. If the fFN is negative, there is a low chance of preterm delivery, given the high negative predictive value of 99.5% for delivery within 7 days. If the fFN is positive, it is less predictive of preterm birth but about 13% will deliver in the next 7 days and nearly half will deliver at less than 37 weeks' gestation.[3] Owing to the possibility of preterm birth, patients should be managed as having a higher risk for preterm delivery.

Management of preterm delivery is gestational age-dependent. Pregnancies less than 37 weeks' gestation can receive corticosteroid injections to accelerate fetal lung maturity.[2] Current guidelines recommend the use of betamethasone or dexamethasone over 48 hours. If the pregnancy is less than 34 weeks, the goal is to delay delivery for at least 48 hours, if the maternal-fetal status is stable, to get corticosteroids on board. Tocolytic agents that can be used are listed below (**Table 6**). If the pregnancy is less than 32 weeks, magnesium sulfate is recommended for neuroprotection of the fetus.

ELECTRONIC FETAL MONITORING

FHR monitoring is commonly achieved with an external fetal monitor and provides valuable information about the fetus' overall health.[4,5] External monitoring is classified according to the following categories.

A category I tracing is normal; therefore, continued monitoring is appropriate. A category III tracing is abnormal and worrisome for the fetus; therefore, delivery should be expedited. The most common category, however, is category II, which involves all other scenarios that do not present in the first and third categories.

Basics of Fetal Heart Rate Monitoring

- Baseline FHR during a 10-min segment rounded to the nearest 5 beats per minute (bpm) increment (normal 110–160 bpm)
  - Bradycardia: less than 110 bpm

Table 6
Tocolytics

Tocolytic	Uses	Side Effects	Contraindications
Indomethacin (COX inhibitor)	Between 24 and 32 wk	>72 h premature constriction of the ductus arteriosus and oligohydramnios	Maternal platelet dysfunction, bleeding disorder, gastric ulcer, liver dysfunction, kidney dysfunction, asthma
Nifedipine (calcium channel blocker)	32–34 wk GA; <32 wk if a contraindication to indomethacin	Nausea, flushing, headache, dizziness, palpitations, tachycardia	Known hypersensitivity, hypotension, or pre–load-dependent cardiac lesions
Terbutaline (beta-agonist)	Second line (Black box warning)	Tachycardia, hypotension, palpitations, tremor, shortness of breath, chest discomfort; hypokalemia, hyperglycemia, and lipolysis; rare myocardial ischemia	Cardiac disease, poorly controlled hyperthyroidism, or diabetes
Magnesium sulfate	Ineffective	Diaphoresis, flushing	Myasthenia gravis, pulmonary edema

Abbreviation: GA, gestational age.

- ○ Tachycardia: greater than 160 bpm
- Baseline variability: fluctuations in FHR greater than 2 cycles per minute
  - ○ Absent: undetectable amplitude range (peak to trough)
  - ○ Minimal: less than 5 bpm
  - ○ Moderate: 6 to 25 bpm
  - ○ Marked: greater than 25 bpm
- Accelerations: abrupt increase in FHR above baseline reaching peak less than 30 seconds
  - ○ Gestation less than 32 weeks: elevation > baseline by 10 bpm for at least 10 seconds
  - ○ Gestation greater than 32 weeks: elevation > baseline by 15 bpm for at least 10 seconds
  - ○ Prolonged acceleration: increase in FHR for 2 to 10 minutes
- Decelerations: decrease below the baseline by 15 bpm for at least 15 seconds
  - ○ Episodic: not associated with contractions
  - ○ Periodic: associated with contractions (early, late, variable)
  - ○ Types of decelerations:
    - ■ Early deceleration: *gradual* decrease in FHR with onset to nadir greater than 30 seconds; occurs at the peak of the contraction
    - ■ Late deceleration: *gradual* decrease in FHR with onset to nadir greater than 30 seconds; onset of the deceleration occurring after the peak of the contraction
    - ■ Variable decelerations: *abrupt* decrease in FHR ≥15 bpm with onset to nadir less than 30 seconds and lasting ≥15 seconds.
- Further classification:
  - ○ Recurrent: occurs with greater than or equal to 50% of contractions in any 20-min segment
  - ○ Prolonged: decrease of ≥15 bpm for greater than 2 min and less than 10 min

Intrapartum Fetal Heart Monitoring

Category I: normal

- Baseline 100 to 160 bpm, moderate variability, ± accelerations, ± early decelerations

Category II: indeterminate

- Tachycardia, bradycardia without absent variability, minimal variability, absent variability without recurrent decelerations, marked variability, no accelerations with stimulation, recurrent variable decelerations with minimal or moderate variability, prolonged decelerations, recurrent late decelerations with moderate variability

Category III: abnormal

- Sinusoidal
- Absent variability with recurrent late or variable decelerations, or bradycardia

Abnormal Fetal Heart Rate Tracings

1. The sinusoidal pattern has a regular amplitude and frequency and appears as a smooth undulating wave lasting for at least 10 minutes. There is a fixed cycle of 3 to 5 cycles per minute.
   a. Management: expedite delivery

2. Decreased variability, either persistently minimal or absent, is the most significant intrapartum sign of fetal compromise. Etiologies include fetal metabolic acidosis, central nervous system depressants such as narcotics and magnesium sulfate, fetal sleep cycles, congenital anomalies, prematurity, fetal tachycardia, preexisting neurologic abnormality
3. Nonreactive FHR tracing (no accelerations).
   a. Absence for more than 80 minutes correlates with increased neonatal morbidity
   b. Fetal scalp stimulation should induce an acceleration; if not, it is worrisome
   c. Causes include hypotension, hypoxia, placental abruption, tachysystole, cord compression, cord prolapse

Interventions for Concerning Fetal Heart Rate Tracings

Category II is an intermediary category that encompasses all the remaining findings not included in category I or category III (see description above). Depending on the fetal heart tracing pattern, select intrauterine interventions can be initiated. For instance, with recurrent variable decelerations, we may try a change in position, intravenous (IV) hydration, and a cervical examination to assess for a prolapsed umbilical cord. (See **Fig 2**)

Intrauterine Resuscitation

Fetal heart monitoring is common in all labor and delivery units, and it is our responsibility to correctly interpret and manage any abnormal findings.[4] Changing maternal position is one of the first noninvasive interventions as umbilical cord compression can cause concerning FHR changes. If there are repetitive decelerations and labor is being augmented with oxytocin, it should be discontinued. Repetitive decelerations can also be a sign of umbilical cord prolapse; therefore, a vaginal examination should be performed. If there is tachysystole (more than 5 contractions in 10 minutes, averaged over a 30-min window) present, then the administration of terbutaline can help relieve frequent contractions. **Fig 3** summarizes these actions. Category 3 tracings are worrisome, and delivery is expedited. Vaginal delivery may be appropriate if the patient is 10 cm dilated and low station; otherwise, an emergent cesarean delivery is indicated.

STAGES OF LABOR
The First Stage of Labor

Defined as the stage from initial dilation of the cervix until complete dilation at 10 cm, the first stage of labor is divided into the latent phase and active phase. During the latent phase, the cervix usually experiences slow cervical change, less than 1 cm of change per hour, due to regular uterine contractions that are intense enough to cause effacement and dilation.

During the latent phase, contractions increase in frequency and typically become more painful, although the intensity varies appreciably. The anatomic uterine divisions of labor become increasingly evident during this phase. The upper segment is firm during contractions, whereas the lower segment is softer, distended, and more passive.[6] Therefore, the upper segment contracts to expel the fetus, whereas the lower uterine segment and cervix dilate and forms a thinned-out tube through which the fetus can pass.[6]

Historically, labor progression was assessed using the Friedman Curve. According to the Friedman Curve, latent labor was prolonged when it exceeded 20 hours in nulliparous women and 14 hours in multiparous women, and active labor began at

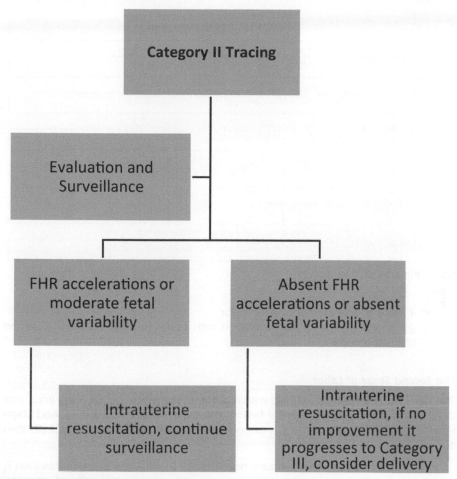

Fig. 2. Management of a category II tracing.

4 cm. More recent data by the Consortium on Safe Labor[7] were used to revise the definition of normal labor, with the active phase of labor starting at 6 cm; the rate of active phase dilation was substantially slower than the Friedman data, varying from 0.5 cm/h to 0.7 cm/h for nulliparous women and from 0.5 cm/h to 1.3 cm/h for multiparous women.

Assessments in the first stage of labor
The cervical examination consists of 5 components assessed by digital examination. The components include cervical dilation, effacement, station, consistency, and position (**Table 7**).

First stage of labor dystocia
Recommendations to prevent primary cesarean delivery have focused on allowing women to labor beyond the historical points established by Friedman.

- Arrest at the first stage of labor: At or beyond 6 cm of dilation with ruptured membranes who fail to progress despite

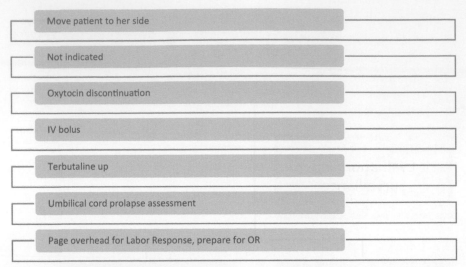

Fig. 3. Intrauterine resuscitation.

- 4 hours of adequate contractions, or
- ≥6 hours of oxytocin administration with inadequate uterine activity and no cervical change

The Second Stage of Labor

Ten centimeters of dilation marks the start of the second stage of labor and ends with the delivery of the neonate. Several factors can delay the length of the second stage including parity, delayed pushing, fetal position, and fetal station. Risks of a prolonged second stage may include:

- Multiparous, greater than 3 hours: neonatal risk 5-min Apgar score of less than 7, admission to the neonatal intensive care unit, and a composite of neonatal morbidity were significantly increased.[8]
- Multiparous, greater than 2 hours: neonatal risk similar to above when the second stage greater than 2 hours.[9]
- Maternal risk: higher rates of puerperal infection, obstetric anal sphincter injury (OASIS), and postpartum hemorrhage (PPH). Also, with each passing hour, there is a progressive decrease in the chance for spontaneous vaginal delivery. Up to 30% to 50% may require operative vaginal delivery.[10]

Table 7 Bishop score[13]				
	0	1	2	3
Dilation, cm	Closed	1–2	3–4	≥ 5–6
Effacement, %	0–30	40–50	60–70	≥80
Station	−3	−2	−1, 0	+1, +2
Consistency	Firm	Medium	Soft	
Position	Posterior	Mid	Anterior	

Second stage of labor dystocia

- For multiparous women, 2 hours of pushing without delivery may be considered abnormal.
- For nulliparous women, 3 hours of pushing without delivery may be considered abnormal.
- Epidural anesthesia or fetal malposition may increase these time frames, but if there is progress in fetal descent, then continued effort should be allowed.

Available techniques to reduce cesarean delivery rates in the second stage of labor

- Operative vaginal delivery (vacuum, forceps)
- Manual rotation of the fetal occiput (preferably with ultrasound guidance)

Common indications for primary cesarean delivery[11]

<• Labor dystocia/arrest (34%)
<• Abnormal or indeterminate fetal heart tracing (23%)
- Fetal malpresentation (17%)
- Multiple gestation (7%)
- Suspected fetal macrosomia (4%)

LABOR AND DELIVERY (L&D)
Induction of Labor

Often, spontaneous labor is not achieved at the time of admission to the L&D unit. Patients who present with prelabor rupture of membranes may require induction of labor. There are several medical indications for a scheduled induction of labor, including hypertension, medication-controlled diabetes, oligohydramnios, nonreassuring fetal status, and post-term pregnancy. Identifying the best available agent to achieve labor progression is crucial. Equally important is identifying conditions where induction of labor is not recommended, including a contracted or distorted pelvic anatomy, abnormal placentation, active genital herpes or cervical cancer, appreciable macrosomia, severe hydrocephalus, fetal malpresentation, and worsening nonreassuring fetal heart tracing.

There are several FDA-approved mechanical and pharmaceutics interventions for induction of labor.[12] Mechanical induction is often achieved with a single or double intracervical balloon. A 30 mL Foley bladder single balloon catheter inserted into the endocervix is commonly used, and commercially prepared double intracervical balloons are also available. Both devices work well to stimulate cervical change. Balloon catheters have minimal side effects and no absolute contraindications. Rare side effects include a prolapsed umbilical cord as fetal head displacement may occur. Also, insertion of a foreign object into the uterine cavity, while the membranes are ruptured, has a potential risk for intraamniotic infection (IAI), therefore, conversation with your patient should occur to discuss the potential risks. Mechanical dilation is thought to work by direct physical pressure on the internal cervical os and by causing the release of prostaglandins from the decidua, adjacent membranes, and cervix.

Medical induction can be achieved with prostaglandin derivatives to ripen the cervix, and oxytocin, to induce or augment labor. Prostaglandin promotes biochemical changes that lead to cervical ripening and myometrial contractility. The prostaglandin E1 analog misoprostol is considered an off-label use but is as effective as the alternatives and has been deemed safe and efficacious by the American College of Obstetrics and Gynecology (ACOG). Misoprostol can be administered vaginally or orally. Regimens vary per institution, but an initial dose of 25mcg is often used; redosing can occur in intervals of 3 to 6 hours.

Prostaglandin E2 analogs include dinoprostone vaginal insert or gel. The vaginal insert is 10 mg of dinoprostone and is FDA approved for cervical ripening. The other option contains 0.5 mg of dinoprostone in 2/5 mL of gel administered endocervically. This dose can be repeated in 6 to 12 hours if there are inadequate cervical changes or minimal uterine contractions, but the maximum dose is 3 doses per 24 hours (1.5 mg). It is important to highlight that prostaglandin should be avoided in patients who have had a previous uterine incision, including a cesarean delivery or myomectomy, due to the risk of uterine rupture.

Oxytocin stimulates uterine contraction by activating G-protein–coupled receptors that trigger increases in intracellular calcium levels in uterine myofibrils and increase prostaglandin production. The synthetic formulation has been used to induce or augment labor since its development in the 1950s.[12] The onset of action is in 3 to 5 minutes, and a steady-state is achieved by 40 minutes. Various titration protocols exist so it is important to follow institutional guidelines.

The Bishop Score[13] is the cervical examination assessment that is predictive of successful induction of labor. It is based on station, dilation, effacement, consistency, and position of the cervix. Although higher Bishop scores are associated with a higher chance of vaginal delivery and lower Bishop scores are associated with a higher chance of cesarean delivery, there is no universally agreed-upon score to identify a favorable cervix. Commonly, a score of 6 or more is considered favorable, whereas a score of less than 3 is unfavorable. If the cervix is considered favorable, administration of oxytocin can begin without a cervical ripening agent.

The combination of an induction agent (prostaglandin, intracervical balloon) with oxytocin does not appear to increase adverse obstetric outcomes and may have a benefit over the use of a single method alone. A meta-analysis of 30 randomized trials showed that a combination of either balloon catheter plus a prostaglandin or oxytocin compared with balloon alone showed a hastened time to vaginal delivery, increased chance of delivery within 24 hours, and did not significantly increase the chance for cesarean delivery or adverse effects.[14]

Other methods of labor induction include artificial rupture of membranes (also known as amniotomy), nipple stimulation, and membrane sweeping. These have variable success rates and should be used at the provider's discretion.

A Failed Induction of Labor

The Consortium on Safe Labor data found that from 4 cm to 6 cm, both nulliparous and multiparous women experienced cervical dilation at the same rate. After 6 cm, multiparous women dilated more rapidly. Data also highlighted that the active phase of labor began at 6 cm when the maximal slope in change occurred. Although this datum is robust, it does not address the management of protraction or arrest of labor.[7]

A prolonged latent phase is defined as greater than 20 hours in nulliparous women and greater than 14 hours in multiparous women. If the maternal and fetal status allows, a longer duration of the latent phase can be allowed and requiring that oxytocin be administered for at least 12 to 18 hours after membrane rupture before deeming the induction a failure. Cervical dilation of 6 cm is considered the threshold for the active phase of labor. Active phase arrest occurs for women at or beyond 6 cm dilation with ruptured membranes who fail to progress despite 4 hours of adequate uterine activity or at least 6 hours of oxytocin administration with inadequate uterine activity and no cervical change.

In the second stage of labor, allowable time for pushing in multiparous women should be 2 hours, and 3 hours in nulliparous women. An additional hour is provided for women with epidural anesthesia or fetal malposition if progress is documented.

Manual rotation of the fetal occiput or operative vaginal delivery can be attempted by a trained provider as an acceptable alternative to cesarean delivery.

The Birthing Process

Once the second stage of labor begins, the cervix is 10 cm dilated and fetal descent has occurred. The fetus is undergoing position changes to accommodate the descent through the birthing canal, known as the cardinal steps of labor (**Fig. 4**). Maternal position during delivery can vary depending on patient and provider comfort and preferences. Upright position increases the pelvic dimensions, improves fetal alignment within the birth canal, increases capacity for pelvic joint movement, and uses gravity's downward force. Often, with epidural anesthesia, positions that require lower extremity strength and sensation should be limited. Supine positions with a lateral tilt are effective as well.

Pushing can also vary between patients as some feel the urge to push and should be encouraged to do so as they please so long as there is a progression of fetal descent and maternal and fetal status are reassuring. Coaching while pushing may occur when patients request guidance or are unable to feel the urge to push due to epidural anesthesia. Often, coaching involves encouraging women to pull their thighs back, tuck their chin to their chest, take a deep breath, and bear down for 10 seconds with 3 repetitions per contraction. Patients should be allowed to rest between contractions.

Episiotomy can be considered for deliveries with a high risk for severe perineal laceration, significant soft tissue dystocia, or to facilitate the delivery of a possibly compromised fetus. Routine use of episiotomy is not beneficial and should be restricted.[15]

Once fetal delivery is imminent, the medical provider's role is to reduce the risks of maternal perineal trauma and fetal injury. Various techniques are used and often depend upon the provider's experience and preference. Controlling the delivery of the fetal head using the provider's hand can be passive or active, particularly during head extension toward the maternal urethra. It is important to encourage only small expulsive efforts when the head is crowning to reduce the chances of injury that

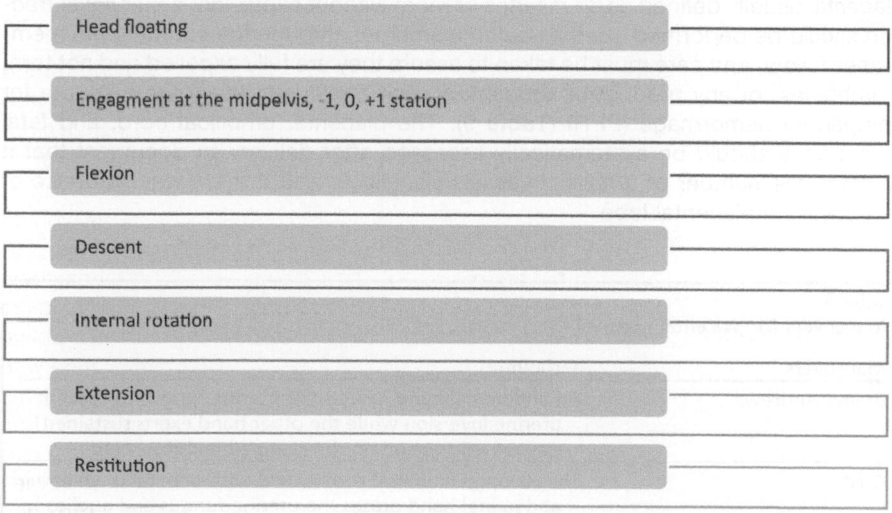

Fig. 4. Cardinal steps of labor.

can occur with rapid expulsion. With one hand guiding the extension of the fetal head, the other hand eases the perineum away from the fetal head and applies a gentle compression pressure. Once the fetal head emerges, fetal restitution will occur. If there is a nuchal cord, it should be manually reduced. A tight nuchal cord can be doubly clamped and cut. Once managed, a hand is placed on each side of the fetal head and gentle downward traction is used to deliver the anterior shoulder. The posterior shoulder is delivered with gentle upward traction. The delivery is complete when the fetal body is spontaneously expelled or with a gentle maternal push.

Skin-to-skin contact and early initiation of breastfeeding (within 1 hour of birth) reduce neonatal morbidity and mortality.[16] Skin-to-skin connection immediately after vaginal birth or cesarean birth leads to more stable vital signs and increased mean blood glucose during the first days of life.[17] Within the first hour of birth, the neonate will initiate the "breast crawl" to find and latch to the breast.

In term infants, ACOG recommends delayed cord clamping for at least 30 to 60 seconds if it does not interfere with the timely care of the newborn or compromise the safety of the mother or baby.[18] The advantage of delayed cord clamping is a higher fetal iron store at 6 months, which is favorable because iron deficiency is associated with impaired neurodevelopment. Disadvantages include hyperbilirubinemia in the immediate newborn period leading to phototherapy use. For preterm infants, the delivering provider should use their judgment with each scenario.

Active Management of the Third Stage of Labor

After fetal delivery, the myometrium thickens resulting in placental detachment due to shearing forces. Signs of placental attachment include a gush of blood, lengthening of the umbilical cord, a firmer and more globular uterus after the placenta detaches, and expulsion. Active management of placental delivery is performed to decrease the risk of postpartum blood loss and the need for a blood transfusion and consists of prophylactic administration of oxytocin before the delivery of the placenta plus gentle traction of the transected umbilical cord and uterine massage. Of note, there are 2 described methods for applying cord traction: the Brandt-Andrews maneuver and the Crede maneuver (**Table 8**). In the event of a retained placenta, usually defined as 30 minutes or more without expulsion, a manual extraction should be performed. As the placenta emerges through the introitus, the membranes follow, and care must be taken to assure they are fully expelled and not torn. Membranes, or any product of conception, that remains in utero are a source for postpartum hemorrhage (PPH) (**Table 9**). The placenta, umbilical cord, and fetal membranes should be systematically assessed after delivery to document that it is intact, the number of umbilical vessels visualized, and if there was evidence of an accessory placental lobe.

Table 8 Maneuvers for placental removal	
Maneuvers	**Technique**
Brandt-Andrews	An abdominal hand secures the uterine fundus to prevent uterine inversion while the other hand exerts sustained downward traction on the clamped umbilical cord
Crede	The clamped umbilical cord is held with one hand while the abdominal hand grasps the uterine fundus and applies sustained cephalad traction

Table 9
Medications used for postpartum hemorrhage

Medications	Dose	Notes
Oxytocin	10–40u in 500–1000 mL normal saline IV or 10 units IM	
Misoprostol	800–1000 mcg PR	Transient fever, nausea, vomiting, diarrhea, headache
Methylergonovine	0.2 mg IM every 2–4 h	Avoid with hypertension
Carboprost	0.25 mg IM every 15–90 min up to 8 doses	Avoid with asthma
Tranexamic acid	1g (10 mL of a 100 mg/mL solution) infused over 10–20 min	

Bleeding after a vaginal delivery should be less than 500 mL. Excessive bleeding most commonly occurs due to uterine atony; however, other causes include lacerations, coagulopathy, or uterine inversion.

Obstetric Complications

Shoulder dystocia
Shoulder dystocia is an obstetric emergency and is identified after the delivery of the fetal head when the anterior shoulder is impacted behind the pubic symphysis. Normally, the fetal bisacromial diameter enters the pelvis at an oblique angle with the posterior shoulder ahead of the anterior one, rotating to an anterior-posterior position at the pelvic outlet with external rotation of the fetal head. The anterior could then slide under the symphysis pubis for delivery. If, however, the shoulders do not descend in this fashion, the shoulder can become impacted, most commonly at the pubic symphysis although a posterior obstruction at the sacral promontory could occur.

Shoulder dystocia should be suspected when the fetal head retracts into the perineum after expulsion, often called the turtle sign. Dystocia is diagnosed when gentle downward traction of the fetal head fails to deliver the anterior shoulder. Common maneuvers used to dislodge the anterior shoulder include the McRoberts position, suprapubic pressure, and delivery of the posterior arm. The McRoberts position is thighs abducted and hyperflexed onto the abdomen. Personnel should be notified of the shoulder dystocia and instructions should be provided including annotating the time, calling for help from anesthesia, pediatric, and obstetric staff. The patient should be encouraged to stop pushing and repositioned to supine with the buttocks at the edge of the bed for optimal access. Laying the patient flat and assuming the McRoberts position helps to increase the anterior-posterior diameter of the pelvic inlet by reducing lumbosacral lordosis which can help dislodge the shoulder by moving the pubic symphysis over the anterior shoulder. If not successful alone, one can ask personnel to apply continuous suprapubic pressure to reduce the diameter of the fetal shoulders to allow the shoulder to slip under the symphysis pubis. If both these maneuvers are unsuccessful, then internal maneuvers should be attempted.

Vaginal access is easier posteriorly with fingers compressed and the thumb tucked into the palm. These maneuvers include delivery of the posterior arm, Rubin's, Wood's screw, reverse Wood's screw, and rotation of the woman onto all fours. Documentation and debriefing are crucial.

Postpartum hemorrhage

In 2017, ACOG revised the definition of PPH to a cumulative blood loss of greater than or equal to 1000 mL or bleeding associated with signs and symptoms of hypovolemia within 24 hours of birth regardless of the delivery route.[19] Common causes include atony, trauma, and coagulopathy. Risk factors include retained placenta or membranes, morbidly adherent placenta, lacerations, large for gestational age neonate, overly distended uterus (ie, macrosomia, polyhydramnios, multiple gestation), leiomyoma, grand multiparity, infection, hypertensive disorders, and precipitous delivery. Management includes early identification and requests for IV hydration, uterotonic medications, and blood products as needed. If lacerations are present and cause excessive blood loss, they should be repaired promptly. Institutional policies on the management of PPH should exist, including escalation to surgical management and appropriate consultations.

Obstetric anal sphincter injury

OASIS is commonly referred to as third- and fourth-degree perineal lacerations. They involve injury to the anal sphincter and the anal mucosa. Proper repair is crucial to avoid wound breakdown and subsequent anal incontinence. Risk factors for OASIS include vaginal delivery, primiparity, labor induction or augmentation, operative vaginal delivery, episiotomy, fetal macrosomia, prolonged second stage, fetal occiput posterior presentation, and increasing maternal age.[15] Preventative techniques include warm compresses to the perineum. Management of an OASIS injury includes surgical repair and postpartum behavioral changes including avoidance of constipation. Surgical techniques consist of a multilayer closure.

- Repair the torn anal mucosa using a continuous (nonlocking) 3.0 or 4.0 braided polyglactin on a tapered needle.
- The internal anal sphincter should be identified and repaired as a separate layer. It often retracts laterally and superiorly and appears as a thickened, pale pink, shiny tissue just above the anal mucosa. A continuous 3.0 polyglactin suture on a tapered needle is used for the repair.
- The external sphincter is then identified and repaired. The ends appear dark red and are grasped with Allis clamps. The repair consists of either an end-to-end or overlapping plication of the ends and its capsule using interrupted or figure-of-eight sutures. Either a 2.0 or 3.0 polyglactin suture can be used.
- Once the sphincter is repaired, the distal rectovaginal septum and perineal body are repaired using techniques for first- and second-degree tears.
- Antibiotic prophylaxis should be administered according to protocol.

Intraamniotic infection and inflammation

Clinical chorioamnionitis or IAI consists of acute inflammation of the membranes and chorion of the placenta. In 2015, a National Institute of Child Health and Human Development Workshop expert panel recommended the use of "triple I" to refer to intrauterine infection or inflammation or both.[20]

IAI is typically polymicrobial but most commonly caused by genital mycoplasmas (Ureaplasma, Mycoplasma). Other pathogens include anaerobes (*Gardnerella vaginalis*, Bacteroides spp), enteric gram-negative bacilli, and group B Streptococcus. Risk factors include prolonged labor and prolonged rupture of membranes. Fever, maternal leukocytosis, maternal tachycardia, fetal tachycardia, uterine tenderness, bacteremia, or purulent or malodorous amniotic fluid are often seen in IAI. The diagnostic criteria are listed in **Table 10**.

Table 10
Intraamniotic infection and inflammation (triple I)

	Fever	Fetal Heart Rate	WBCs	Amniotic Fluid
Presumptive Diagnosis:	Fever 102.2 F once or 100.4 F to 102.2 on 2 or more measurements	Baseline fetal heart rate >160 bpm for 10 min or more, excluding accelerations, decelerations, and marked variability	Maternal WBC count >15,000 ideally showing a left shift (absence of steroid use)	Purulent appearing amniotic fluid via speculum
Confirmed Diagnosis:	All of the above (fever, tachycardia, elevated WBCs, purulent amniotic fluid) *plus*: 1. Amniotic fluid with: • Positive Gram stain of amniotic fluid • Low glucose level in amniotic fluid • Positive amniotic fluid culture *or* • High WBC count 2. Histopathologic evidence of infection or inflammation or both in the placenta, fetal membranes, or the umbilical cord vessels			

Abbreviation: WBC, white blood cell.

Management includes antibiotic therapy, antipyretics, and delivery. Broad-spectrum antibiotics should be administered at the time of diagnosis. If Intrapartum, the current suggested regimen is ampicillin 2g IV every 6 hours plus gentamicin 5 mg/kg IV once daily.[21] If a cesarean delivery is initiated, the addition of clindamycin 900 mg IV every 8 hours is added. Institutional guidelines should be followed.

Indications for cesarean section
Some conditions warrant a cesarean delivery for the safest outcome, such as the accepted indications for cesarean deliveries as well as the selective indications (**Table 11**).

Trial of labor after cesarean/Vaginal birth after cesarean
Trial of labor after cesarean (TOLAC) occurs in patients with a prior cesarean delivery and, after appropriate consultation, desire a trial of a vaginal delivery. Counseling

Table 11
Indications for cesarean section

Accepted	Selective
Failed IOL	Breech presentation
Cephalo-Pelvic disproportion	Repeat cesarean
Failure to dilate	Major congenital fetal anomalies
Fetal distress	Cervical cancer
Placental abruption	Prior surgical vaginal repair
Placenta previa	Large vulvar condylomata
Cord prolapse	HIV infection
Active HSV infection	
Conjoined twins	

Abbreviations: HIV, human immunodeficiency virus; HSV, herpes simplex virus; IOL, induction of labor.

regarding the optimal mode of delivery depends on the patient's preference, obstetric history, previous vaginal births, and reason for previous cesarean delivery. Vaginal birth after cesarean (VBAC) calculators from the Maternal-Fetal Medicine Units Network (MFMU) are available to calculate the likelihood of success. Risks of TOLAC include uterine rupture with a need for hysterectomy, infection, and perinatal mortality. Optimal candidates include those with only 1 to 2 previous low transverse cesarean deliveries, particularly when the previous cesarean delivery was not due to failure to progress, and those with a history of a vaginal delivery. VBAC is a vaginal birth after cesarean and is the desired outcome for patients undergoing TOLAC.

CLINICS CARE POINTS

- Reducing the number of primary cesarean sections for nulliparous term singleton and vertex pregnancies is ideal due reduce the complications of cesarean section.
- If the opportunity to perform a trial of labor safetly, then it should be discussed with the patient and plan should be put in place for the best outcomes.

DISCLOSURE

The authors have nothing to disclose.

REFERENCES

1. In: Cunningham F, Leveno KJ, Bloom SL, et al, editors. Obstetrical Hemorrhage. Williams Obstetrics, 25e. McGraw Hill. Available at: https://obgyn.mhmedical.com/content.aspx?bookid=1918&sectionid=185083809. Accessed August 18, 2021.
2. Management of preterm labor. practice bulletin No. 171. american college of obstetricians and gynecologists. Obstet Gynecol 2016;128:e155–64.
3. Rapid fFN® for the TLiıQ® System. Information for health care providers. Hologic 2020. Available at. https://www.hologic.com/package-inserts/diagnostic-products/ffn-test. Accessed September 2021. URL.
4. Intrapartum fetal heart rate monitoring: nomenclature, interpretation, and general management principles. ACOG practice bulletin no. 106. american college of obstetricians and gynecologists. Obstet Gynecol 2009;114:192–202.
5. Management of intrapartum fetal heart rate tracings. Practice Bulletin No. 116. American College of Obstetricians and Gynecologists. Obstet Gynecol 2010;116:1232–40.
6. Cunningham F, Leveno KJ, Bloom SL, et al, editors. Physiology of Labor. . Williams Obstetrics, 25e. McGraw Hill. Available at: https://obgyn.mhmedical.com/content.aspx?bookid=1918&sectionid=185083809. Accessed August 18, 2021.
7. Safe prevention of the primary cesarean delivery. obstetric care consensus no. 1. american college of obstetricians and gynecologists. Obstet Gynecol 2014;123:693–711.
8. Cheng YW, Hopkins LM, RKJr Laros, et al. Duration of the second stage of labor in multiparous women: maternal and neonatal outcomes. Am J Obstet Gynecol 2007;196:585.e1-6.
9. Allen VM, Baskett TF, O'Connell CM, et al. Maternal and perinatal outcomes with increasing duration of the second stage of labor. Obstet Gynecol 2009;113:1248–58.

10. Rouse DJ, Weiner SJ, Bloom SL, et al. Second-stage labor duration in nulliparous women: relationship to maternal and perinatal outcomes. eunice kennedy shriver national institute of child health and human development maternal-fetal medicine units network. Am J Obstet Gynecol 2009;201:357.e1-7.
11. Barber EL, Lundsberg LS, Belanger K, et al. Indications contributing to the increasing cesarean delivery rate. Obstet Gynecol 2011;118(1):29–38.
12. Induction of labor. ACOG practice bulletin No. 107. american college of obstetricians and gynecologists. Obstet Gynecol 2009;114:386–97.
13. BISHOP EH. Pelvic scoring for elective induction. Obstet Gynecol 1964;24:266–8.
14. Orr L, Reisinger-Kindle K, Roy A, et al. Combination of Foley and prostaglandins versus Foley and oxytocin for cervical ripening: a network meta-analysis. Am J Obstet Gynecol 2020;223(5):743.e1–17.
15. Prevention and management of obstetric lacerations at vaginal delivery. ACOG practice bulletin no. 198. American college of obstetricians and gynecologists. Obstet Gynecol 2018;132:e87–102.
16. Optimizing support for breastfeeding as part of obstetric practice. ACOG committee opinion no. 756. american college of obstetricians and gynecologists. Obstet Gynecol 2018;132:e187–96.
17. Moore ER, Bergman N, Anderson GC, et al. Early skin-to-skin contact for mothers and their healthy newborn infants. Cochrane Database Syst Rev 2016;11: CD003519. Accessed August 26, 2021.
18. Delayed umbilical cord clamping after birth. ACOG committee opinion No. 814. American College of Obstetricians and Gynecologists. Obstet Gynecol 2020; 136:e100–6.
19. Postpartum hemorrhage. practice bulletin No. 183. american college of obstetricians and gynecologists. Obstet Gynecol 2017;130:e168–86.
20. Higgins RD, Saade G, Polin RA, et al. Evaluation and management of women and newborns with a maternal diagnosis of chorioamnionitis: summary of a workshop. Obstet Gynecol 2016;127(3):426–36.
21. Intrapartum management of intraamniotic infection. committee opinion no. 712. american college of obstetricians and gynecologists. Obstet Gynecol 2017; 130:e95–101.

Moving?

Make sure your subscription moves with you!

To notify us of your new address, find your **Clinics Account Number** (located on your mailing label above your name), and contact customer service at:

Email: journalscustomerservice-usa@elsevier.com

800-654-2452 (subscribers in the U.S. & Canada)
314-447-8871 (subscribers outside of the U.S. & Canada)

Fax number: 314-447-8029

Elsevier Health Sciences Division
Subscription Customer Service
3251 Riverport Lane
Maryland Heights, MO 63043

*To ensure uninterrupted delivery of your subscription, please notify us at least 4 weeks in advance of move.